CONCEPTS OF CARE: DEVELOPMENTS IN HEALTH AND SOCIAL WELFARE

Edited by

Richard Hugman BA, CQSW, PhD

Professor of Social Work, Curtin University of Technology,
Perth, Australia

Moira Peelo BA, MPhil, PhD

Honorary Research Associate, Lancaster University,
Lancaster, UK

Keith Soothill BA, PhD

Professor of Social Research, Lancaster University,
Lancaster, UK

A member of the Hodder Headline Group
LONDON • SYDNEY • AUCKLAND

First published in Great Britain in 1997 by
Arnold, a member of the Hodder Headline Group,
338 Euston Road, London NW1 3BH

Whilst the advice and information in this book is believed to be true and
accurate at the time of going to press, neither the authors nor the publisher
can accept any legal responsibility or liability for any errors or omissions
that may be made.

British Library Cataloguing in Publication Data
A catalogue record for this book is available from the British Library

Library of Congress Cataloging-in-Publication Data
A catalog record for this book is available from the Library of Congress

ISBN 0 340 65254 3

Typeset in 10/12pt Palatino by Phoenix Photosetting, Chatham, Kent
Printed and bound in Great Britain by JW Arrowsmith Ltd, Bristol

Contents

List of contributors

Stephen Ackroyd
Professor of Organisational Analysis, Management School, Lancaster University, Lancaster, UK, and an organisational consultant

Shaheen Azmi
Doctoral Graduate, Faculty of Social Work, University of Toronto, Toronto, Canada

Rosalie A. Boyce
Research Fellow, Graduate School of Management, University of Queensland, St Lucia, Brisbane, Australia

Gracy Fernandes
Research Director, Research Unit, College of Social Work, University of Bombay, Bombay, India

George Giacinto Giarchi
Emeritus Professor of Social Care Studies, Department of Social Policy and Social Work, University of Plymouth, Plymouth, UK

Richard Hugman
Professor of Social Work and Head of the School of Social Work, Curtin University of Technology, Perth, Australia

Graham B. McBeath
Senior Lecturer in Sociology, Department of Sociology, Nene College of Higher Education, Northampton, UK

Kalindi Mazumdar
Honorary Professor, College of Social Work, University of Bombay, Bombay, India

Maggie Pearson
Professor and Regional Director of Research and Development, NHS
Executive, North West Regional Office, Warrington, UK

Moira Peelo
Honorary Research Associate, Department of Applied Social Science,
Lancaster University, Lancaster, UK

Ann Pursey
Assistant Professor, Department of Nursing Studies, University of Hong
Kong, Hong Kong

Deborah Quinney
Research and Development Facilitator at the Worcestershire Community
Healthcare NHS Trust, Worcester, UK and Associate Fellow at the Centre for
Health Services Studies, Warwick Business School, Warwick University,
Coventry, UK

Keith Soothill
Professor of Social Research, Department of Applied Social Science,
Lancaster University, Lancaster, UK

Stephen A. Webb
Head of Communication and Information Studies, University of North
London, UK

Introduction

1

Boundaries of care – an introduction

Richard Hugman, Moira Peelo and Keith Soothill

Why boundaries of care?

Ideas about 'care' and 'caring', and the social practices to which they relate, are, at a surface level, commonsense notions. This is an important aspect of the general human condition, one which may be said to be a marker of civilized life. Our societies may be analysed in relation to the extent that they succeed or fail in exhibiting this attribute. At the same time 'care' has a 'homely' quality that embodies a positive sense of the human condition at a particular level. Individual people as well as whole societies can be understood in these terms. Because it is such an embedded commonsense term, it is widely used in the English-speaking world in ways which simply relate approval, acceptance or positive regard.

Why, therefore, a book to examine thought and practice in health and social welfare concerning this concept? There are, we suggest, two principal reasons why such an analysis is pertinent. First, scholarship in the last decade increasingly has identified the importance of this topic for understanding the structures and practices of health and social welfare services. Of specific concern has been the interrelationship of different aspects of society, namely the person, the family, the community (or neighbourhood) and the state (Finch, 1989; Ungerson, 1987). Within such studies social relations at each of these various levels have been identified as crucial to a recognition of 'care' as a key element in the construction and reconstruction of contemporary identities (for example, concerning gender). Who we are and how we live is defined at least partly in terms of 'care'.

Second, the nature of health and social welfare services in themselves have been developed around claims to the expression of caring at the social level. Welfare states have come to be seen as 'the caring society' in action, so that the public provision of health and welfare is axiomatic with claims to 'caring' (Barry, 1990). Attempts to redefine the structures and practices of welfare states therefore become highly contested, precisely because they go to the heart of what is valuable in our societies and valued in ourselves – they challenge notions of the 'good' which are communicated through the idea of care.

In both these respects there is now a major reappraisal and restructuring of welfare states in progress on a global scale (Evers, 1993). In the 'advanced' industrial countries where welfare states had become established over much of the twentieth century there has been a move away from a single-sector perspective to one which recognizes the plurality of stakeholders in the definition and practice of caring (Bartlett and le Grand, 1993; Svetlik, 1993). The separation of private and public expressions of care and caring has been replaced by models which seek to address the connections between different sectors, including the state, various types of non-government agencies (for-profit and not-for-profit) and the 'informal' sector (families and neighbours). Such diversity introduced potential competition into claims to care, as each sector defines it in relation to itself. In this sense the so-called 'advanced' countries are 'catching up' with the rest of the world where less fully developed state sectors have meant that plurality has been more widely recognized for longer (cf. Midgley, 1981). To identify the boundaries of care, and the changes to which they are subject, a range of possible interpretations must be considered.

Approaches to care

Mayeroff (1972, p. 2) proposed that distinctions should be made between caring for a person and caring for an idea. While each may combine aspects of personal action and intellectual and emotional attachment, there is a difference of balance between the two which renders it necessary to make a distinction. However, there are common links insofar as the quality of 'caring' is to be found in a commitment towards the protection, growth and development or achievement of potential of the other person or the idea (pp. 10–12). This commitment may be both abstract (as in thought) and concrete (as in action). For Mayeroff, caring is also to be found in the personal characteristics (intellectual and emotional) of the person who cares: in the possession and use of knowledge; in moral values (such as honesty); or in personal traits (such as patience) (pp. 13 ff., 28 ff.).

The distinction between ideas and people as the objects of caring has been developed in feminist scholarship, particularly within analyses of the ways in which this concept has affected the lives of women (and some men) through recent social policies and the practices of health and social care professions. This analysis is marked by its separation of thought and emotion from action. Graham (1983) has delineated between caring as emotional and intellectual commitment (love), and caring as the performance of tasks that enable another person to live (labour). Ungerson (1983) similarly distinguishes between caring *about* and caring *for*. The importance of these distinctions is to note that ideas and actions in caring can be separated practically as well as analytically. The person who performs a caring task may or may not have the accompanying emotional or intellectual commitment to the object of their care. Indeed, it is an important aspect of 'informal' care, demonstrated through empirical research, that people who 'do' caring may well not 'feel' caring (Finch, 1989; Hicks, 1988; Ungerson, 1987).

Mayeroff conceived of caring as the connection between thought and action. It has been suggested that in some respects Mayeroff's argument may be tautological (Hugman, 1991, p. 10). The example given was that of a father who goes in the night to fetch a doctor for a sick child. Mayeroff argues that the father 'does not experience this as a burden; he is simply caring for the child' (1972, p. 9). If the father, experiencing a burden, did not go, then to say he was uncaring would produce a circular argument, or at least be seen as self-evident. Moreover, such a distinction assumes that purity of motive both defines the subsequent action and its degree of caring – neither of which is actually necessary nor allows for the ambivalence and contradictions of human existence. So, for example, what of the father who does experience this as a burden, but who goes anyway? This is the situation evident in the lives of people quoted by Ungerson (1987) and Finch (1989). Such a position would appear to be more a contradiction in terms, if our understanding of care depends only on Mayeroff's connection between thought/feeling and action.

There is a moral ingredient in popular assumptions about care, by which it is seen as an individual's expression of love and concern; compulsion negates the expectation that care is about personal involvement which is freely given, whatever the work conditions. Within the world of paid work this 'individual contribution', which turns acts of care into something to be valued, is expressed in the language of 'vocations' and a drive to express one's individuality through a specific profession. In this way, the feminist analysis exposes the extent to which caring practice cannot be used in a simple way as a measure of social values. If one has no alternative but to undertake certain tasks for another, then this cannot be an expression of the 'good' either in relation to oneself as a person or of the society in which one lives (Davis and Ellis, 1995). In the language of moral philosophy, the degree to which one is compelled to 'do' caring (by custom, by social pressures or by the lack of alternatives) is inversely related to the extent to which one 'is' caring. Caring as an ethical position or value cannot exist without choice; there is no virtue in being compelled. To this extent understanding the concept of care is, therefore, to grasp a contradiction.

Care in context

Each of these concepts of 'care' is rooted in an historical context, with beliefs grounded in the political and economic reality of any given time and place. It is difficult to conceive of practices or policies which might exist in an abstract dimension without historical analysis. To some extent there is an apparent divide between the public and private spheres in theorizing about care which is communicated through giving primacy to care within the context of informal networks (family or kinship, friendship, neighbourliness). In some instances this divide is more a matter of perspective, developed to enable social policy to be examined through an empirically grounded critique of contemporary circumstances. At the same time, however, the divide between public and private is not always quite as clear or as obvious as might at first appear to be the case. Indeed, Simmel (1955) saw the human capacity for individuality as predicated on industrial society's fragmentation, allowing one person to belong to numerous groups – individuality being the sum of cross-cutting allegiances and cross pressures meeting in one person. Recent debates have focused on this point at which social forces and sentiments meet, through attention to the relationship between the personal and the political dimensions of people's lives. Attention has been given to the 'informal' sector and to those people who use health and social care services to balance an earlier neglect of their circumstances and interests.

Yet within the wide-reaching changes taking place in the way care and caring are socially structured and expressed there are professional groups for which the question of the meaning of care also is important (Hugman, 1991). These are the practitioners in health and social care whose work produces those services which constitute the formal or public sphere whether state, for-profit or voluntary. The role of the voluntary sector specifically concerns the bridges between the two spheres, and the interweaving of beliefs, values and individual choices in social action. For this reason, we are concerned in this book to address recent analysis of the conception, development and implementation of any manifestation of what might be seen as 'public care'. This will, of necessity, involve attention to the historical and political dimensions of 'care' as well as the contemporary policies and practices through which it is manifest in the public sphere. By political and historical context we mean that our understanding of the intention and impact of the public provision of care cannot be a philosophical or scholastic debate alone. Although an examination of the philosophical underpinnings of policy and systems helps us to understand more deeply how a specific system evolved and what various sub-plots there may have been (albeit without awareness on the part of the instigators) such an approach does not inform us of the narrative of implementation or of the gulf between political rhetoric and reality of provision. This requires a more detailed empirical inquiry.

Historical and political dimensions to care

In the UK the 'welfare state' has a central place in the post-war world of building 'a land fit for heroes'. Although key elements of public welfare (such as old-age pensions) pre-date this, the post-war period saw the institutionalization of welfare as public caring in a variety of state agencies. A comparable situation can be seen throughout Europe, although the specifics differ between countries (cf. Esping-Andersen, 1990). The impact of the 1939–45 war on individuals' knowledge, through army experience, work experience, travel and a breakdown of other networks, released the necessary atmosphere to enact changes already long considered in the pre-war years of the nascent British Labour Party. The ideas may not have been entirely new but the political conditions needed to make real those ideas had arrived. At the same time, the mainland of Europe was, perforce, undergoing rebuilding and regeneration in response to quite particular post-war conditions. As well as rebuilding bombed cities and relocating and rehousing the vast numbers of displaced persons, post-war Europe was subject to enforced ideologies of de-nazification as well as the occupation of the new communist bloc. Victorious allies imposed central control for all aspects of society, from education to government, in West Germany; Western Europe gained from the Marshall Plan, but US generosity was shaped by a fear of insurgent communism, particularly in France and Italy (Hennessy, 1992, pp. 297–8). Eastern Europe was adjusting from war and German occupation to communist control. What all had in common was an enforced need for government intervention through rationing, through regeneration and through defeat, of most areas of life, including provision of basic food, education, housing policies and minimal health care. Although state provision was patchy, depended on local conditions and may have been temporary in nature, it nonetheless marked a sea change in how governments defined their roles.

In the UK, the new post-war Labour government was clearly elected to establish state provision of care: the electorate of 1945, as Taylor has pithily summarized, cared for their own future housing, full employment and social security (1975, p. 723). However, the fortunes of the new welfare state were dependent on the economic strength of a small island of limited international power, whose condition in 1945 has been described by Hennessy as 'morally magnificent but economically bankrupt' (p. 94). The United Kingdom no longer benefited from its old colonial role, it had few natural resources and it had not recovered from the nineteenth century depression which had undermined the old, heavy industrial base. The sudden removal of wartime financial agreements (Lend–Lease) by the United States on 21st August 1945 threatened to destroy what economic resources there were. Moreover, old colonial allegiances were finally blasted apart by new world orders that were ultimately demonstrated when, much later, OPEC flexed its muscles and started to charge competitive rates for oil in the 1970s.

Public care in the contemporary era

War, as an agent of social change, is powerful, but also demands pragmatism of politicians. It reminds governments of the need to have a fit population sufficiently educated to make sense of machinery, arms and instructions. Once the memory of war has passed, so too does the sense of urgency and the concern for the welfare of pregnant women, babies, children and potential soldiers fades into the background. They become seen as humanitarian concerns, luxurious worries which, 40 years or more after the formation of welfare states, are increasingly seen as a series of private, consumer choices rather than a matter of legitimate concern for government (Evers, 1993). In such circumstances concern for public care becomes highly contested (Barry, 1990). It can now plausibly be represented as unwarranted interference of the state in an individual's private concerns, while at the opposite end of the spectrum the view that state care is a humanitarian imperative, necessary to show that one's political entity has ethical underpinnings, also remains but with less force than previously.

Both extremes of the debate and their philosophical concomitants weigh more or less heavily on the see-saw of provision according to the economic and political fortunes of time and place. Somewhere in the middle is written the narrative of the reality of public provision: surviving the rough times, embodying the accommodations of the previous period and attempting to meet the needs of the present time. These are the circumstances in which health and social care professionals currently find themselves.

Seeking to ground our discussion within its historical and political context is not to return to a positivist, empiricist position versus an interpretation of phenomena. As we have noted above, this implies no claim to the universality of certain truths about the nature of public care. Nor is there any suggestion of an 'historicism' which would argue that with the passage of time some teleological, historical imperative of progress has moved us forward to the development of public care, or that the whole job of historical change has been to produce, inevitably, the structures of this moment. Rather, it reflects the belief that political action affects, for good and ill, the tenor of ordinary people's lives and that political praxis embraces the range of social life. This can be seen both in the 'everyday' choices of action through which society routinely is reproduced, or it can be found at the extremes. This is illustrated by the (former) German terrorist Bommi Baumann, who said that

> Political practice doesn't have to be terrorism, it can be anything – even daycare, things like that. But we just happened to be active in that area. We saw it as political work inside the total framework (1977, p. 38).

Baumann shocked fellow travellers in a statement about the need, ultimately, to choose between love and terrorism. This may be seen as a move from one expression of 'care' to another (although he did not use such terms). As a pre-echo of the feminism which was to follow him, rather than choosing either politics or individual relationships he might have recognized that 'the personal is political'. Individual relationships, the voluntary giving of love or labour and care within the family (the economic unit of love) support and maintain the labour force and connect the private sphere to the public sphere. The arbitrary divide between private and public enables us to sidestep questions concerning the extent to which personal experience is individual and unique, or shaped and warped by larger forces. For 1960s urban guerillas there was no doubt: private choices were political actions, hence shoppers and workers injured or killed in bombed department stores were not innocent bystanders; in addition, they saw individuals as subjugated to a capitalist system through 'an illusion of contentment by the material plenty' (Becker, 1978, p. 38). So by attacking apparently personal aspects of life, political activists felt they made individuals aware of the social dangers inherent in apparently private choices.

The Red Army Faction's belief in the guilt of consumerism echoes Marcuse's view that the liberating potential of technology has been subverted by 'voluntary servitude' as capitalism engenders a need in people to own and possess gadgetry of all kinds, hence 'the majority of organized labour shares the stabilizing, counter-revolutionary needs of the middle classes, as evidenced by their behaviour as consumers of material and cultural merchandise' (1969, p. 24). The material and cultural merchandise consumed includes health and housing, food, educational qualifications and personal care. The technology of health has expanded exponentially in the post-war period, raising expectations of disease-free longevity unanticipated in the pre-war era. At least into the 1960s this was accompanied, in the more developed industrialized countries, by an expansion of public services, predominantly state-sector or state-supported, which were held to be universal in their benefit and therefore the achievement of a caring society.

However, the New Right thinkers of the 1970s and 1980s might agree with Marcuse that 'social morality is rooted in sexual morality' (1969, p. 18), as they subsequently began to (re)place the responsibility to care not in the public arena but within the home and the biological family (cf. van Every, 1992). Care, when located in the private sphere, is imbued with a voluntarism that triggers associations with 'natural' families, with private choices, with a sexual division of labour. Within the private sphere care is redolent of wealth, consumerism and right-thinking choices – the 'naturalness' of love is biological and bounded by notions of duty and kinship (for a fuller account of this debate, see Abbott and Wallace, 1992). Within the public sphere all that can be described as best can also be viewed as worst, a contradiction which O'Brien tackled in his pithy word-portrait of Schweitzer, who has stood as a symbol of altruism and self-sacrifice in the eyes of a white public, whereas 'To educated Africans and Afro-Americans . . . he represents the most irritating, if not the most noxious, aspects of the white man in Africa: paternalism, condescension, resistance to change' (1965, p. 289).

The above example illustrates the limitations of unregulated voluntarism. Class differences, race differences, caste differences and gender differences in who receives and who gives such 'public' care and the question of who needs most versus who benefits most, raise issues of internal colonialism within a given state as well as issues of cultural and professional imperialism (Midgley, 1981). That very embodiment of goodness is, paradoxically, its essential badness: that care is arbitrarily accorded to the lucky few who happen to be within the orbit of the individual who has chosen to give generously that which, by definition, belongs to them to give. It is not under the control of the receiver nor is it freely accessible to the receiver, but dependent on the will, judgement and generosity of one person who has the power whimsically to withdraw what is needed should he or she so decide.

So, under these circumstances, the will to implement defeat of the 'five giants' remains the property of the powerful as does the capacity to be free of hunger, disease, ignorance, poor housing, poverty and want. The needy still do not have, as their own right or property, good health, good nutrition, housing, education, etc. For that they remain dependent on internal colonialism, on the philosophy and will of others at a given point in time to focus what resources exist to alleviate the suffering in the lives of fellow citizens. Suffering is transformed into a private sorrow; alleviation of need outside the bounds of one's family and kinship system must be explained and accounted for on a public stage. The particular, the personal, is, in effect, shared experience acted out in isolation. What interest, then, can the social polity have in breaking that isolation? What is the role of the health and social welfare workers within structures that do not presuppose their services as underpinned by minimum rights but, at least philosophically and politically, as a charitable service or else a consumer good?

Caring (and the) professions

Throughout the history of the welfare state the professions have played a central role. Not only have they been the vehicle through which policy has been implemented in practice, but also their skills and knowledge frequently have come in many instances to be synonymous with the alleviation of health and welfare problems. It has been observed that the very nature of professionalism is often, for these occupations, interwoven with claims to 'caring' as one of its core features (Hugman, 1991). The professional, it is asserted, is someone who through their skilled and knowledgeable practice demonstrates commitment to the person (as an individual) and to the goal of helping (in general). Some professional groups even have used the notion of 'love' in their public statements about their identity and objectives (Hugman, 1991, p. 18). 'Caring' can define some professionals, and a 'duty of care', as a bureaucratic tool, can define others; but 'care' can also be used to define boundaries between the duties of workers and professionals working closely in similar institutions. Witz (1992) has cogently argued that male medical practitioners combined to ensure control of diagnosis and treatment of illness within the public sphere (in particular, see Chapter 3 on 'Gender and medical professionalisation'), allowing the tending of the sick, and all that entails, to women at home and female nurses in hospitals. Although nursing and medical practice is no longer so sharply gendered in its division of labour, there are still different sets of expectations surrounding the duties of each group, even if both are perceived as committed to the health of patients. The nature of the care from different professionals can be quite specifically defined by the caring acts expected: although not all health and welfare professions perform basic labour in aspects of daily living, such as bathing, toileting and so on, they do all share claims to the degree of commitment that we discussed above. Commitment of this kind may be seen in many ways, such as a willingness to deal with issues that others do not consider, being available when needed, showing the qualities (described by Mayeroff, 1972) of patience or compassion, and so on.

It is this factor (a mixture of personal qualities and commitment) in concepts of care which is expected to transcend work conditions and duty, that part of vocation which cannot be bought, that element of goodwill which expresses an individual's caring. So the doctor who insists on going home at 5:00 p.m. when there are still patients to see will, by definition, be seen as uncaring, as will nurses or social workers who engage in industrial action such as strikes. (Insofar as this latter action would be seen as caring it would, we suggest, for many people be on the same terms as the terrorist discussed above.) Mackay (1993) argues that, in the case of nurses, vocation implies 'a quiescent and submissive stance: they are there to serve others' (p.51) and that, unlike police and firefighters who exchanged 'no-strike' agreements for index-linked salaries, nurses are still expected to put patients first without such pay rewards.

Nonetheless, once a vocational choice is made, professional decisions are fraught with an ethical dilemma: that in many situations 'caring' actions defined in this way (commitment and personal qualities) may be seen simply as the person 'doing their job'. If without freedom of action there is no virtue, can the performance of such work be considered as 'caring' at all? While an individual professional may be allowed the notion of 'vocation' as a generalized explanation for the choice of paid career which allows open expression of care and concern beyond immediate pay and conditions, there has been increased use of the idea of a 'duty of care'. This duty often falls on an agency, and responsibility is bureaucratically apportioned with agreed protocol for professional action. Apart from statutory responsibilities, the growth of procedural correctness is well illustrated throughout UK government 'Health of the nation' publications; and, while protecting professionals against litigation, such correctness assumes the needy and client groups to be without responsibility. While, of course, an agency may have a duty of care, it is individual workers who are culpable. How, then, can the content of care work, which is highly personal or interpersonal, be separated from ideas about 'care' in academic analysis, professional self-images or even in the public consciousness? How are such issues addressed in thinking about policy or the organization of formal services? It is these and related questions with which this book is concerned.

This book

We are primarily concerned with the public sphere in this volume. The chapters which follow all begin with the public arena. This includes three sectors: the state sector; for-profit services; and 'voluntary' services (that is the not-for-profit sector) (Svetlik, 1993). The fourth sector, of 'informal' care, that we have referred to above as the 'private sphere', in some ways cannot be separated from the others. Increasing attention is being paid in social policy to the ways in which these four sectors form a 'welfare mix' (Evers, 1993). Within the 'welfare mix' the 'informal' sector is a major element. However, as we have noted above, much has been written in recent years that exposes the private sphere to public scrutiny. Attention to the public sphere has either been from the perspective of overall policy or else has tended to focus on the minutiae of practice. While each of these is important, there has been little debate at the middle level to examine the impact of recent changes and developments on the formation of caring in the public sphere.

The following chapters examine a range of issues. The organization of caring services, their location within the state, the nature of professionalism in caring work, the connections between caring and community and the very ideas and social structures around which these institutions and practices are constructed have in recent times been subject to changes which are both far-reaching and rapid. To chart these changes and to explain them is an enormous task. In this collection we make a contribution to such an exercise, aware of the limitations that any one book must necessarily possess. However, the structure of this volume and the topics covered within it, we contend, do define important areas in which this subject can be explored as well as identifying key themes for the analysis of caring as an organized public activity.

In Part 1 theoretical and conceptual issues are examined. In Chapter 2 Ackroyd looks at the recent history of state welfare and questions the widely held assumption that the welfare state is a response to the fear of social unrest. Insofar as the welfare state can now be seen as being in decline in Western society, the evidence of widespread unrest and opposition is curiously lacking. The relationship of the state, society and formal care has shifted dramatically, so that other areas of life have now replaced welfare as the location of such negotiations between states and citizens (cf. Barbalet, 1996). In Chapter 3 McBeath and Webb approach this point from the perspective of thinking about postmodernity and the way in which the sites of caring have moved and fragmented. The social class analysis which underpinned earlier understandings of social welfare as a response to the demands of citizens must be seen as cross-cut by questions of other social divisions such as gender, race and culture, sexuality, disability and age. Debates around these different, sometimes competing, discourses contribute to the critique and reappraisal of social welfare that results, in part, with attempts at the privatization of care.

Part 2 examines empirically recent developments in formal care services. In Chapter 4 Quinney *et al.* look at community nursing in the UK and the construction of the professional self-identity of the community nurse around the notion of caring work. Challenges to the boundaries between nursing and other professions are seen as a major feature of recent restructuring of health and welfare. In these circumstances care is both commitment to service and (often) sheer hard work, but is also reflected in the definition of nursing itself as an holistic enterprise. The nature of nursing is defined in terms of care as the integration of 'labour' and 'love'. Likewise, in Chapter 5 Boyce examines the impact of health-services' restructuring on allied health professions (otherwise known as 'ancillary to medicine') in Australia. There are strong elements of similarity in the developments in the two countries, with comparable impact on professional identities of 'caring' professions. In both these chapters the boundaries of care as a set of tasks and as a set of professional commitments are seen to be shifting as relationships between the state, the professions and service users change rapidly.

In Part 3 two 'non-Western' views of care are presented in explorations of social work in Canada and India. In Chapter 6 Azmi analyses the meaning of care for traditional Muslim communities in Canada, concluding that concepts of 'professional imperialism' (cf. Midgley, 1981) are inadequate. Instead, Azmi proposes an understanding of social work as a modernist enterprise which is missionary in character when applied to traditionalist communities. This is a reading of social work which resonates with the analysis of Parton (1994) that social work's modernist claims to 'care' are at best partial. Transcultural application of such practices may be limited, at best, because the modernist discourse of social work does not connect to the religious and cultural assumptions of 'traditionalism' and at the same time does not always acknowledge its own connections to social control. In contrast, in Chapter 7 Fernandes and Mazumdar discuss the developing meaning of care within social work in India. This example illustrates the impact within Eastern culture of a profession with clear roots in Western society. What is seen is the absorption of social work and its refocusing through the cultural and social lens of India. In this context the parallels and similarities between East and West are seen to be greater than the distinctions. Together the chapters in Part 3 indicate boundaries not only of formal care in relation to non-Western cultures but also of debates about post-colonialism as a defining aspect of cultural difference in care. These are both voices of 'otherness' in 'Eurocentric' professional discourse, but at the same time they also make statements of clear difference, pointing to a rich global diversity (Thrift, 1993).

The fourth and final part of this book examines contemporary issues in care. In Chapter 8, in a discussion of European developments, Giarchi argues that the grasp of social divisions in formal care practices is the major factor in European social welfare. In particular, he examines the notion of discrimination and its converse expressed in 'antidiscriminatory practice'. This is seen as foundational to social welfare in the late twentieth century. In Chapter 9 Peelo takes a complementary stance, identifying the role of 'voluntary' caring as an important ingredient in the development of social welfare. While critical of the concept of the 'active citizen', she nevertheless shows that the activity of citizens cannot be divorced from an understanding of care policies and practices. Indeed, it is a lack of such analysis that leads governments to misunderstand the choices made by individual citizens to express their commitment in this way. Such an understanding points to the ambiguous nature of community, which is also identified by Hugman in the final chapter. He reviews the critiques of the notion of community and its application to care, looking at the importance of social divisions (especially around gender and 'race') for a more pertinent grasp on the realities of care. It is only if this is done, he argues, that the connections between community as place and as people, and between care as task and sentiment, can be used as a vehicle for the construction of new forms of social welfare.

Through the different parts of this book the reader is invited to consider the ideas, structures and practices that constitute formal care and the changes to which they are subject. We have not attempted to propound a unitary line of argument but to reflect diversity and debate. However, there are two underlying issues which each chapter addresses in some way. First, developments in policy and practice that fail to understand the complex reality of caring and the interrelationship of state, professions and community are unlikely to succeed in their own terms; such approaches will leave a legacy of unintended consequences. Second, that the nature of care cannot be analysed without reference to social divisions reflects the divided global and local societies in which we live; recognizing and challenging such divisions is a crucial part of the caring responsibilities of the state, the professions and communities. While the reader is invited to draw her or his own conclusions, the evidence presented here is that the boundaries of care continue to shift, marking a major element in the shaping of future patterns of social welfare.

References

Abbott, P. and Wallace, C. 1992: *The family and the New Right*. London: Pluto Press.

Barbalet, J. 1996: Developments in citizenship theory and issues in Australian citizenship. *Australian Journal of Social Issues* **31**(1), 55–72.

Barry, N. 1990: *Welfare*. Buckingham: Open University Press.

Bartlett, W. and le Grand, J. 1993: The theory of quasi-markets. In le Grand, J. and Bartlett, W. (eds), *Quasi-markets and social policy*. Basingstoke: Macmillan. 13–34.

Baumann, B. 1977: *How it all began: the personal account of a West German urban guerilla*. Ellenbogen, H. and Parker, W. (trans). Vancouver: Pulp Press.

becker, j. 1978: *Hitler's children: the story of the Baader-Meinhof Gang*. London: Panther Books.

Davis, A. and Ellis, K. 1995: Enforced altruism in community care. In Hugman, R. and Smith, D. (eds) *Ethical issues in social work*. London: Routledge. 136–54.

Esping-Andersen, G. 1990: *The three worlds of welfare capitalism*. Cambridge: Polity Press.

Evers, A. 1993: The welfare mix approach. Understanding the pluralism of welfare systems. In Evers, A. and Svetlik, I. (eds) *Balancing pluralism*. Aldershot: Avebury. 3–32.

Finch, J. 1989: *Family obligations and social change*. Cambridge: Polity Press.

Graham, H. 1983: Caring: a labour of love. In Finch, J. and Groves, D. (eds), *A labour of love*. London: Routledge and Kegan Paul.

Hennessy, P. 1992: *Never again: Britain 1945–51*. London: Vintage Books.

Hicks, C. 1988: *Who cares?* London: Virago.

Hugman, R. 1991: *Power in caring professions*. Basingstoke: Macmillan.

Mackay, L. 1993: *Conflicts in care*. London: Chapman & Hall.

Marcuse, H. 1969: *An essay on liberation*. London: Pelican.

Mayeroff, M. 1972: *On caring*. New York: Harper & Row.

Midgley, J. 1981: *Professional imperialism: social work in the Third World*. London: Heinemann.

O'Brien, C.C. 1965: *Writers and politics*. London: Penguin Books.

Parton, N. 1994: Government, (post)modernity and social work. *British Journal of Social Work*, **24**(1), 9–32.

Simmel, G. 1955: *Conflict and the web of group affiliations*. London: Glencoe.

Svetlik, I. 1993: Regulation of the plural and mixed welfare system. In Evers, A. and Svetlik, I. (eds), *Balancing pluralism*. Aldershot: Avebury. 33–50.

Taylor, A.J.P. 1975: *English history 1914–1945*. London: Pelican.

Thrift, N. 1993: The light fantastic: culture, postmodernism and the image. In Clark, G.L., Forbes, D. and Francis, R. (eds), *Multiculturalism, difference and postmodernism*. Melbourne: Longman Cheshire. 1–21.

Ungerson, C. 1983: The language of care. In Finch, J. and Groves, D. (eds), *A labour of love*. London: Routledge and Kegan Paul.

Ungerson, C. 1987: *Policy is personal*. London: Tavistock Publications. 31–49.

van Every, J. 1992: Who is the family? The assumptions of British social policy. *Critical Social Policy* **11**(3), 62–75.

Witz, A. 1992: *Professions and patriarchy*. London: Routledge.

Part 1: Theoretical and conceptual issues

Editors' introduction

Examining theoretical and conceptual issues can seem daunting, but it is crucial to try to understand what underpins our notions of care and caring. Reflecting on a period of quite remarkable change in social welfare provision in many countries, a sense of a break with the past is often to the fore. However, as Ackroyd stresses in Chapter 2, 'concepts of social care display remarkable continuity' (p. 19). He argues that a particularly important theme has been the positive social effects of provision. At a time when variants of state welfare provision are under challenge, he reminds us how social care may contribute to social integration and so, in turn, to social order. In brief, social care is held to be important – by adherents to very different political doctrines – to the development of a unified and effective society. Within a theoretical context which sees social care as functional, Ackroyd suggests that 'the failure to provide for adequate social care could well have explosive results not presently envisaged by policy makers' (p. 32). What this means is that the provision of only meagre levels of social care may have quite devastating social effects. Whether Ackroyd's 'strong' thesis will come to pass may be questionable, but there is no doubt that we need to face the potential consequences of changes in welfare provision.

McBeath and Webb make an especially focused theoretical interpretation of recent developments in community care in the UK which they see as part of a broader political strategy of a government pursuing what has been termed a 'New Right' agenda. However, the success of the shift in political terms would have been unlikely without a clever fusing of left radicalism with right libertarianism. Together they have heralded the retreat of the interventionist state and so provided the opportunity for the reappearance of a doctrine of civil society. In brief, community care can be identified as an attempt to reallocate responsibilities from the public sector to voluntary associations, to the market and to families.

Although much used, 'care' is a curiously elusive concept. Indeed, as McBeath and Webb stress, what care is in terms of conceptual analysis has been neglected. They make a bold attempt to fill this gap. Essentially they are recommending that we can begin to grasp contemporary usages and practices of care when we appreciate how a discourse of care has actually emerged in modern Western societies. In emphasizing the importance of specific historical and social contexts, they also provide a useful theoretical foundation for the explorations of 'non-Western' views of care which follow later in Part 3.

2

Don't care was made to care

Stephen Ackroyd

Functions of social care?

In Britain the need for social care has been advocated as part of some very different political doctrines, yet concepts of social care display remarkable continuity. One central and recurring theme which will be considered in this chapter concerns ideas about the positive social effects of provision. Social care is seen not just as an obligation of the privileged towards the less privileged, still less is it seen as a moral absolute, as something rewarding or virtuous in its own right. It is characteristic for British ideas about social provision to have a utilitarian and even a functional cast. Ideas about social care have tended to suggest that care is valuable because of what it contributes to society. Specifically, it is held to contribute to social integration: care supposedly contributes to social order and to the development of a unified and effective society.

Functional ideas about care have been a feature of right-wing thinking as much as liberal and left ideas. Traditional right-wing doctrines have always tended to be organicist and nationalistic. 'Old Tory' conservatism, with its emphasis on 'natural' hierarchy fits well with ideas of self-regulating community and the value of an integrated society (Beer, 1965). To this way of thinking, basic social stability is the foundation on which economic prosperity at home and any successful territorial expansion of Empire is necessarily built. From this it is inferred that it is sometimes necessary to build national solidarity and, should it fail to emerge automatically, to develop institutions which will secure integration. Such is the character of the paternalistic 'Old Tory' attitude to social care. It is less fully appreciated that a similar sort of rhetoric was used to justify both social liberal and reformist socialist ideas about social care in the nineteenth and early twentieth centuries. Social liberalism, for example, draws attention to the destructive social effects of the decay of community caused by the extension of markets. Material and, even more so, cultural impoverishment produces alienation and the decline of identification of people with the community as a whole (Sabine, 1951). The route back to an effective society is therefore through the agency of institutions designed to reintegrate and to re-engage the citizenry. Only slightly less extreme in its stress on paternalistic themes, the Fabian socialism which was so important in developing the practical ideas for the administration of the welfare state shared many points of agreement with this basic logic of national efficiency. The route to social efficiency is by effective integration of society through appropriate national institutions (McBriar, 1962).

In short, whether we consider ideas about social care expressed in traditional Toryism beginning in the eighteenth century, social liberalism first devised in the middle nineteenth century, reformist 'Fabian' socialism of the early twentieth century or even the Butskellite consensus over the welfare state in the early post-Second World War period, a common theme of otherwise quite different doctrines is that social provision promotes social harmony and contributes positively to a unified society. Indeed, it is possible to go further and assert that British ideas about social care have typically been interwoven with nationalism. An effective society, it is argued – by Tories, liberals and socialists alike – is one integrated by institutions designed for the purpose. Further, on the occasions the country has faced military and economic threats, effective social care has been identified as a means to integration. So the provision and extension of social services has been recurrently promoted by the discovery that the country had been ill-prepared for war. Similarly it is suggested that social care may help a country to compete effectively in economic arenas. Hence, social care is supposed to provide a sense of national identity and solidarity. In this sort of way, provision for social care is held to contribute directly to social and economic effectiveness.

The broad base of agreement in British political thought about the need for social care helps to explain the secure basis on which the welfare state was founded in the decade following the end of the Second World War. Ideologically, the welfare state secured some support from all classes. This helps to explain the extent of the support for the institutionalization of social care. Against a background of economic and political instability, and in recognition of a need for a huge effort to restore national effectiveness in the immediate post-war period, the appeal of the functional view of social care was irresistible. In brief, the welfare state was set up not only to secure health, education and social security provision, but also because it was thought to contribute to social solidarity and integration. For many it was the foundation of a new social contract and a secure basis on which to re-establish Britain as a world power. The lynchpin of this consensus was the peculiarly British idea of citizenship which was held to guarantee political *and* social rights (Marshall, 1950, 1977; Turner, 1986, 1990, 1993).

Preliminary argument and evidence

It is possible to probe and test the proposition that social care is functional. However, as the effects of social care on social integration which the political philosophy reviewed above envisages are likely to be general and to be manifest over relatively long periods of time, the argument will, of necessity, be historically based. Interestingly, while it is difficult to think of unambiguous indicators of positive social integration, there is a good deal of data and writing concerning the opposite – of social and economic conflict. Hence it is possible to look at the connections between levels of welfare provision and the incidence of various types of socio-economic conflict. The most disadvantaged people in the population have always expressed their discontent in a number of ways – most obviously in forms of overt protest and dissent. These various expressions of conflict – including such things as rebellions, riots and strikes – have been amply studied by specialists. In recent times statistics on such things as levels of state expenditure and strikes have also been available in great abundance. These data have been extensively analysed, not only for Britain but for many other countries.

In principle, it is not difficult to see why social welfare provision might yield social integration. The points to note are that the recipients of welfare will be both materially more secure and feel themselves to be valued. Provision of unemployment insurance obviously has direct economic value. In addition, most services – such as health care or education – may also be seen as having economic value. Services may be viewed, therefore, as redistributing wealth in the population and as having the effect of making people less vulnerable to the vagaries of employment markets. However, the value of social care is arguably more basic than this material contribution because it provides people with a sense of identity and self-worth. As the theory of citizenship states, access to social benefits is a sign that the person receiving them has value (Marshall, 1950; Turner, 1986). In both material and symbolic aspects, then, the provision of social welfare attacks at the root of the basic sources of the feelings of insecurity and injustice that give rise to protest and dissent.

It will be argued from the available literature that, when it is provided, social care can and does contribute to social order and so to lower levels of such things as popular protest and rebellion. Evidence for general relationships between welfare expenditure and the reduction of conflict can be identified in the statistics for a range of Western societies. In the late 1970s, for example, Hibbs (1978) published work which shows graphically the general relationship between welfare provision and strike action. In common with a number of other writers, Hibbs accepted the importance of examining long periods of historical time when looking for connections between state provision and social effects. Hibbs's work considers the relationship between strike incidence and welfare expenditure by comparing data for the period 1910–40 with those for the period 1950–70 over a range of countries. Hibbs took as his measure of unrest a single index of strike activity, which he called strike volume. Using this measure applied to data from eleven countries, Hibbs shows an impressive correlation between the change in the incidence of strikes between the pre-war and the post-war periods and change in the size of state expenditure on non-military services – that is, on the welfare state.[21] This work suggests there was in fact, until the mid-1970s anyway, a fairly precise, linear relationship between the level of expenditure on the welfare state and the level of social unrest as measured by strike activity. According to Hibbs's data, the higher the expenditure on welfare payments made by the state, the lower the levels of strike action in the post-war period were likely to be.

On closer examination, however, the connection between welfare provision and social peace is less straightforward than Hibbs's work implies. Being so general and relating to such long periods of time, Hibbs's work necessarily glosses over important differences between countries, especially in the manner and extent to which the assimilation of conflict has been achieved. It can be argued that there is a direct causal relationship between welfare provision and levels of unrest only at the extremes of state expenditure. It seems that very high levels of welfare provision can substantially guarantee socio-economic peace. Countries that exemplify a strong relationship between high state provision (as measured by state expenditure on services) and high social integration (as measured by persistently low incidence of strikes) do exist in the shape of Sweden and Austria. The reverse also tends to be true: states which spend very little on welfare provision, such as the United States, show recurrent socio-economic unrest which is sometimes primitive and explosive. However, for the middle ranges of state expenditure per capita it is much less clear that the connection between these variables is uniform and direct. Hence, though it is the case that social care is an antidote to unrest, it is important to explore this relationship more fully. In some countries – Britain would be a good example – it can be argued that conflict has persisted at relatively high levels despite the development of a broad spectrum of social welfare provisions.

In this chapter, it will be argued that there are two features which need to be taken into account when considering the positive social functions of care. One is the absolute level of social provision, the other is the timing of the introduction of social provision and the effects of this on public action and sentiment. It is suggested that relatively modest provision of care at a time of acute social need will be more effective in developing social integration than more generous state provision late in the day. Hence it is possible to identify different sequences of development of welfare provision. On the one hand, modest welfare provision that is appropriately timed can lead to social care being seen as functional in securing social integration. On the other hand, if developments in social care are slow to arrive, they may not be very effective in limiting and redirecting well-established tendencies to protest and to take action, so challenging the supposed functionality of the social welfare system. Britain is an example of the latter type of process in the evolution of welfare systems. The funding of the social care system, with the possible exception of the two decades following the Second World War, has never been generous. Furthermore, it was introduced at a very late stage in Britain's political and economic development. For both these reasons the development of the British welfare system did not contribute significantly to the reduction of overt conflict. The lessons to be drawn from this, against the trend of fashionable thinking, are twofold: first to recognize the need for more resources to be pledged to social care and, second, for those resources to be used to better effect.

The main focus of this chapter is to try to understand the process by which British society has accommodated and institutionalized conflict, and the way that social care has (or has not) affected that conflict. The institutionalization of conflict has its roots in the very beginning of economic development and continues until the present time. Hibbs's and other comparable research gives some insight into just part of what is a much longer sequence of change. Since 1975 in Britain, for example, industrial unrest in the form of strikes has unexpectedly declined to the point at which, in 1995, it was at the lowest level since statistics were first collected in the late nineteenth century. Since the mid-1970s also, levels of welfare expenditure have been capped or actually cut, with considerable consequences for expressed conflict.

In analysing historical trends used as a basis for interpreting contemporary change, four stages of institutionalization will be distinguished. The first is the period up to around 1870, when insurrection and riot were as prevalent as striking. The second is the period 1870–1940, in which striking emerges as the single most significant form of protest. This form of protest is securely institutionalized and consolidated by a range of political institutions in the form of various trade unions and links to the polity, but not so far that other forms of protest are entirely eliminated. On the contrary, in this period, other forms of popular protest, among them rioting, continued to exist. They have two patterns: either rioting and so on exist as adjuncts to the strike or they exist as alternative ways of expressing dissent. Third, there is the period 1940–75, in which striking is consolidated as the main form of effective protest but in which the strike takes on its most limited and institutionalized form. In this period too the alternative forms of protest continue to survive. The final period is 1975–95. Against this background of earlier British history, the novel features of this period can hardly be more strongly emphasized and will be discussed in the conclusion to the chapter.

From rebellion and riot to the strike

A key difference between the industrial development of Britain and some other European countries is the length of time that dissenting behaviour provoked by the rise of capitalism was in existence before the achievement of a highly centralized state apparatus, let alone any very extensive welfare system. The contrast between Britain's experience in this respect and that of 'second wave' industrial powers such as Sweden, Germany and Austria is marked (Kemp, 1969; Trebilcock, 1981). For these states, industrialization was achieved to a considerable extent by state sponsorship from the top down, rather than, as in Britain, as a spontaneous development from the bottom up. This is not to say that industrialization was not accompanied by conflict in other countries, because it was. Industrial relations in Sweden were extremely violent in the first two decades of the twentieth century, for example. However, in contrast to Britain, by the fourth decade of the twentieth century, following the adoption of programmes of reform and the election to office of a reforming leftist party, Swedish strike levels began a secular decline from which they have never recovered. Serious conflict did not have a chance to become institutionalized. By contrast, in Britain there was more than a hundred years of unregulated industrial development before the emergence of effective trade unions. Here there was considerable opportunity for forms of violent dissent and protest to emerge and to develop into semi-institutionalized forms.

Historians who have studied collective violence and insurrection during the past three hundred years or so have concluded it is not random. Indeed, public protest and popular disturbance have been shown to exhibit some distinctive patterns. The study of these events – such as riots, demonstrations and rebellions – has also led to the conclusion that this behaviour is not irrational – it usually embodies deliberate intent and has discernible objectives. Because it is motivated, and also usually resisted and opposed, protesting behaviour has adopted distinctive forms which it is reasonable to identify as quasi-institutions. It is in the character of such events that they are, almost by definition, indications of the breakdown of public order, and therefore to describe them as institutions would seem to be at least questionable. However, even riots, which are supposedly instances of massed humanity out of control, have been shown to have recurrent features and typical targets. For all their violence, such events also embody and express desires for positive change and improvement on the part of their perpetrators. These events are motivated by and express moral concern and, though this often fails to be acknowledged, they embody an interest in establishing a different order of things.

Once they have become customary, patterns of behaviour, whether they express solidarity or dissent as in the riot, are slow to change. This persistence as recurrent behaviour is in fact the way we recognize institutions. Yet the partially institutionalized nature of dissenting behaviour took a long time even to be recognized, let alone to be seriously studied. It was not until well into the twentieth century that ordinary people became recognized as a suitable subject for historical writing at all (Cole and Postgate, 1938). Not until after the Second World War was there much attempt to consider 'unorganized' dissenting and protesting behaviour. By the early 1960s, however, a group of historians in Britain began to focus on the behaviour of the 'crowd' and the 'mob'. The first generation of post-war historians of popular dissent and protest (Hobsbawm, 1968; Thompson, 1968) not only recognized that the behaviour of people took customary and quasi-institutionalized forms, but also suggested a general pattern of change in their organization could be identified. The change was labelled by these writers as a transition between 'pre-industrial' and 'industrial' forms of protest (Thompson, 1968). Hobsbawm (1968) used the distinction between 'primitive' and 'modern'. For these writers, popular disturbances (which were frequently violent) in the late eighteenth and early nineteenth centuries in Britain were mostly localized, lacking formal organization and backward-looking in terms of their aspirations. They were overwhelmingly spontaneous protests about the loss of customary benefits and/or the removal of traditional rights. At this time, rioting – motivated by protests over the price of bread or the lack of availability of work, or against conscription or new forms of taxation – was the dominant form of disturbance. Protest was against change, especially change towards market relations and aimed at restoration of customary exchanges. By the end of the nineteenth century, by contrast, disturbances had taken on a quite different motivation, being much more clearly economically motivated, and were concerned with imposing some order and control on new arrangements. Protest had become specifically targeted at gaining and protecting new economic benefits.

For these early analysts, their ideas about motivation also explained a general transition in the dominant forms of protesting behaviour that were adopted. Strike activity, which itself became increasingly organized and focused as the nineteenth century progressed, was a more modern and less primitive form of activity. Although for a long time supplemented by other and quite distinct kinds of behaviour, especially rioting, striking became much the most frequently used type of action as time passed. For these early writers, whereas rioting was the central form of protest in the eighteenth century, the strike had become dominant by the start of the twentieth. The nineteenth century can therefore be looked upon as a transitional period in the predominant form of protest to be observed. In these circumstances it is quite easy to view violence as essentially a passing phase, as the strike itself was usually non-violent and even non-confrontational. Almost by default, therefore, there is a tendency to assume the long-term disappearance of violence, to see it as something that would eventually entirely disappear in the modern period. Yet such an idea is certainly arguable. In fact, the capacity for violent protest runs as a continuous thread through the social history of Britain.

The institutionalization of striking

Writing about conflict in Britain, Cronin (1979) has suggested that striking became slowly but quite definitely differentiated from rioting and insurrection during the nineteenth century. According to him, by the end of the third quarter of the nineteenth century, the strike had been turned into something new and distinct:

> It is clear, then, that strikes became differentiated from earlier forms of collective action only slowly, and even in the nineteenth century the separation has been at certain moments precarious. . . . Nevertheless, there is some consensus that the strike became the 'natural' response to distress in England some time between 1850 and 1900. . . . the break appears sharpest before and after 1870. . . . However, the dynamism of protest did not diminish once the transition from the old to the new forms was accomplished (p. 46).

For Cronin there is also a clear implication that once the 'modernization' of protest had been accomplished, there would be no turning back. For him, in the twentieth century, the study of strikes can be equated with the study of industrial conflict as such. One problem of this sort of position is that it takes no account of the existence or significance of other forms of dissenting behaviour – both behaviour of a 'primitive' kind, such as rioting, and behaviour of even more focused and specialized forms of misbehaviour than striking, such as work limitation and absenteeism. Cronin appears to overlook the possibility that striking came to be the most common form of protest only because of specific historical conditions and that it would cease to be so if these conditions were to change.

In contrast, other writers have been less convinced about the exclusive importance of striking and are much more circumspect when it comes to interpreting the extent to which protest has become permanently transformed and 'modernized'. Charles and Louise Tilly, who have been among the most energetic and gifted of the second generation of students of popular protest, have identified the period 1830–1930 as the 'rebellious century' (Tilly *et al.*, 1974). Their focus of concern is not just Britain but much of Western Europe as well, and they argue for and illustrate great and continuing diversity in the forms of conflict displayed in many European countries. It is their view that, at any point in time, people will have available to them a range of ways of expressing and representing grievances, and many forms of behaviour are potentially available for use. The range of behaviour institutionalized will change only quite gradually, but will continue to be a range. Charles Tilly (1981) suggests that European populations have always displayed what he identifies as distinctive 'repertoires of collective action':

> In Western Europe, the prevailing eighteenth century repertoire differed significantly from the modes of collective action Europeans employ today. Its most dramatic and recurrent forms were the food riot, concerted resistance to

conscription, organised invasions of fields and forests and rebellion against tax collectors. . . . The repertoire which came to dominate the nineteenth century looked quite different. Its most visible collective forms were the demonstration, the protest meeting, the strike, the electoral rally. These are essentially the means by which Europeans today air their grievances (p. 19).

Although Charles Tilly has spent a good deal of time studying the incidence of strikes *per se* as well, with another collaborator (Shorter and Tilly, 1974), the Tillys are not wholly committed to the idea that there is an exclusive form of protest in any period, and for them the option of many forms of protest is permanently available.

However, it is clear that the work of the majority of the social historians suggests the importance of striking as a form of popular protest through much of the twentieth century in almost every advanced country. If one has to settle on a single indicator of popular unrest for much of the twentieth century – as evidence of the lack of effective social integration – then striking is undoubtedly the best candidate. The centrality of strikes as a form of protest is to do with their effectiveness. As the early historians of protest perceived, the strike is partially effective in limiting the vulnerability of people to developing labour markets. While strikes typically make demands on particular employers, and to that extent they embody focused demands, they may be, if appropriately organized, very effective in more general ways. Strikes may be developed into the vehicle for the expression of general economic and political discontents and will be effective in resolving these if they are accompanied by higher levels of institutionalization in the shape of trade unions and political programmes. Because of this, various writers have interpreted the development of strike activity in the present century as being directed towards and culminating in the achievement of political influence as a result of institutionalization (see especially Shorter and Tilly, 1974). The argument has been specifically applied to Britain by Cronin (1979). These writers point to the waves of strike activity, rising over periods of two decades or more during the late nineteenth and early twentieth centuries, which culminated in the achievement of new levels of both trade-union organization and political acceptance of their political programmes.

Returning to the question of whether the provision of social benefits is a significant causal factor in the reduction of social conflict, however, it has to be assumed that the introduction of social care provisions by conservative groups (as was the case in Imperial Germany at the end of the nineteenth century) will be as effective as when they are introduced by left parties. To pursue the issue of the social effectiveness of care, it is necessary to focus in more detail on the development of conflict in Britain and the way that the introduction of welfare provision may be causally related to it. As might be expected, the limited development of social care before the Second World War had little effect on the emerging pattern of socio-economic conflict. Conflict had a developmental pattern of its own, with the obvious tendency during the first three decades of the twentieth century towards increase rather than diminution.

It is important to be clear what is being contended here. Before the Second World War, strikes in Britain were, although the predominant form of protest, relatively infrequent. This was true especially for the period between the two world wars. This was partly because unemployment was generally high, and, in the absence of comprehensive welfare, the costs of a lost job were likely to be considerable. On the other hand, conflict was, by any other standard, extremely serious. Strikes involved very large numbers of people and could well continue for long periods of time. The appropriate image of the strike during that period is as a trial of strength. Confrontations between protesters and the forces of law, when they occurred, could well be bloody. Strikes were protracted and could also involve confrontations with authority, rioting, protest marches and other forms of demonstration. The event which symbolizes conflict at this time in the popular imagination is the General Strike of 1926. In many ways this event was atypical; indeed it can usefully be regarded as a turning point after which the aims of conflict were less overtly political and the demands for reform less total. On the other hand, the way the General Strike combined political and social unrest is not misleading as a symbol of the characteristics of the period.

Conflict and the welfare state in Britain

In an impressive review of the evidence relating to strike activities in thirteen Western countries, Shorter and Tilly (1974) show, in a similar way to Hibbs, that there are different patterns in the incidence of strikes between the pre- and post-Second World War periods. They also found that for some countries industrial conflict withered away in the longer term whereas there were others where the level of strike activity, however measured, remained very high. Britain belonged to an intermediate group of countries in which some reduction in the incidence of conflict was discernible.

Shorter and Tilly's study provides more data than does Hibbs's and allows more subtle interpretation of what has happened. On the basis of Shorter and Tilly's data, the era of the establishment of the welfare state, following the Second World War, was associated with a change in the overall character and objectives of striking. Both the size of strikes (as measured by the average number of participants) as well as their typical length (measured by the average duration of strike events) greatly declined. Certainly, the popular image of industrial conflict in this period that strikes were narrowly instrumental, being focused on wage issues rather than political principle, is borne out by these data. The typical strike involved quite small numbers who were willing to strike only for a short period. Obviously this popular image contains significant elements of distortion as well. Widespread changes in the management and utilization of labour at this time caused considerable and acute reactions from labour.

Be that as it may, there are some grounds for thinking that the deployment of the welfare state by the first majority Labour government (1946–51) took much of the moral and political sting out of industrial conflict at least for the 1950s and 1960s. It now seems clear that the political aspirations that had been associated with striking in earlier decades had by then almost entirely disappeared. In fact, even though the strike persisted as the predominant form of popular protests in post-war Britain until 1980, it had become thoroughly domesticated. Institutionalized conflict in the shape of the small-scale, short-lived strike can be seen as part of a broad pattern of accommodation to conflict – what has been called the post-war 'settlement' between capital and labour (Jessop, 1979). This concept of settlement explicitly refers to an established condition of exchange between the property-owning class and the organized working class. In the British settlement, then, among other things, the management of the economy and the provision of security of employment, including adequate social care, had been exchanged for political quiescence. However, what was distinctive about the situation in Britain was the willingness for organized labour to continue with strikes.

In some crucial respects, however, events do not fit snugly into this view of a stable and managed socio-economic system based on an agreed and effective settlement. One ominous feature was that new forms of politicized protest were evident from an early point – so-called 'race riots' undertaken by disadvantaged elements of the population not in the ranks of the organized working class. The 1950s were thus marked by the rediscovery of some elements of the Tilly's 'repertoire' that had been thought to be forgotten. The capacity to riot by disadvantaged communities in the inner cities is simply the reseparation of the repertoire of forms of conflict. Unlike the pattern of some countries, where strike action went into secular decline after the achievement of social reform, this did not occur in post-war Britain. The long-term general trend of strike activity was upward rather than downward. Trade-union membership burgeoned during the 1960s and 1970s. There were periodic surges of industrial conflict in which the numbers of strikers per strike, in particular, dramatically increased. It is possible to talk of the gradual repoliticization of striking throughout this period. For commentators of left and right this period is seen as rising to a climax in the so-called 'winter of discontent' (1978–79) in which a Labour government had presided over a seemingly endless series of pulverizing strikes. The period had seen the partial rediscovery of the protracted trial of strength, particularly in evidence in the first miners' strike of 1974–75.

It is difficult to correlate variations in the development of the welfare state with variations in overt conflict very precisely. There was a general rise in the funding of social care in the post-war period until the mid-1970s. Government figures show that expenditure rose from just under 15 per cent of gross domestic product (GDP) in 1960 to around 25 per cent of GDP in 1975 (an increase of 66 per cent). Therefore, increasingly generous provision seems to accompany a period of intensifying conflict. However, as has been remarked, British welfare provision was never generous at the best of times and was under considerable strain from competing demands by 1970. Welfare expenditure in Britain certainly did not match the levels of increase undertaken by other states, where industrial peace was more successfully maintained. So, for example, Sweden increased expenditure in the same period from around 16 per cent of GDP to more than 33 per cent (a proportionate increase which had more than doubled). France made a similar scale of increase, and West Germany moved from around 20 per cent of GDP to 33 per cent. Whilst the latter was a similar scale of increase as that in Britain, the increase began from a much higher base. In fact, during this period, Britain barely maintained its relative rank in the top 50 per cent of advanced countries in terms of the size of its expenditure on welfare. At the same time, too, the redistribution of wealth involved in the provision of services was doing little to affect the escalating inequalities of income and life chances in the country at large. The universalistic pattern of service provision favoured in Britain meant that services often were less redistributive than those of many other countries. However, this is not evidence that social care was not functional in Britain, as is now widely believed. It is more accurate to say that welfare expenditure was not as functional as it might have been, and as it was elsewhere in Europe.

Don't care was made to care

Functional ideas about the effects of care have always been contested. Standing in opposition to ideas about the need to provide basic social and economic support for citizens has been the doctrine of the free market and the minimal state. This alternative to the thesis of the functional welfare state achieves precise expression in particular doctrines: economic as distinct from social liberalism and in new conservatism as distinct from Old Toryism. In short, the idea that social care has social functions has been consistently contradicted by ideas which privilege the market. According to these ideas, only individual efforts can and should secure whatever individual welfare there is to gain. With this approach, of course, the invisible guiding hand of the market is thought not to require amendment or direction as a mechanism of distribution. Thus, the best possible outcome to the arrangement of social affairs is allegedly secured by the 'unfettered' working of economic relations and unimpeded freedom of contract. At their most extreme, such views deny the importance of community and can even involve the denial of the existence of anything beyond the contracting individual. Margaret Thatcher's notorious statement 'there is no such thing as society' is a well-publicized recent endorsement of this thesis (on the difference of this position from the majority of Western political theory, see Kingdom, 1992).

On the basis that the social ideals of the welfare state are in error and that the working of markets needs to be re-established, the post-war settlement has been deliberately disrupted in the last two decades of the twentieth century in Britain. From the election of the Conservatives in 1979, the willingness of government to take responsibility for managing the economy, especially in such 'corporatist' directions as overseeing investment levels and guaranteeing full employment, has dramatically declined. Further, there was a sustained assault on the limited control of labour markets that trade unions had established. In a series of measures – no less than nine major pieces of legislation were passed limiting trade union powers between 1979 and 1993 – the powers of organized labour were progressively and systematically reduced. In 1994 the OECD compiled an index of employment security and protection in the advanced countries. Britain was ranked at zero on this index, the lowest of any European country (OECD, 1994).

Partly because of the withdrawal from economic management and partly because of massive underinvestment in production by private industry (Coates, 1994), by the mid-1980s unemployment began to mount to levels unknown since before the Second World War. Hutton (1995), in his recent analysis of the British situation in the post-war period, has stressed how official unemployment figures have been massaged so as to appear less dire and has identified no less than 30 changes being made to the definition of unemployment in recent years (p. 35). Despite difficulties in measurement, recent decades have seen the creation of a form of structural unemployment hitherto unknown. These changes are now identified as an emergent new mass of the permanently unemployed labelled as 'the underclass' (Smith, 1992). Hutton estimates that as many as 30 per cent of the adult population constitute a class of permanently disadvantaged people in the population:

> Altogether some twenty eight per cent of the adult population are either unemployed or economically inactive. Add to this another one per cent who are on government schemes to alleviate unemployment, and the proportion living on the edge is close to one third (1995, p. 106).

The underclass, of course, does not include the large numbers in the employment market now self-employed or with part-time or temporary jobs on the periphery of the economy whom Hutton identifies as in some potential jeopardy.

Despite the marked increase in the numbers of potential recipients of income support, quite remarkably the overall level of expenditure on social security remains at around 22 per cent of GDP. At the very time that government began to withdraw from directing the economy and so allowing unemployment to burgeon, it also embarked on a programme of limiting welfare budgets and reducing the overall level of welfare expenditure. In the years of rising unemployment in the 1980s, the overall level of state welfare expenditure was progressively cut from around a quarter of GDP in 1982, to around a fifth in 1988 (Hills, 1993). As we have seen, the funding of social care in Britain has been in relative decline compared with other advanced countries since the Second World War. Since 1975, this trend has accelerated. Whereas in 1960 Britain's expenditure on the welfare state as a proportion of GDP was just in the top 50 per cent of advanced countries, by 1990 it was in the bottom 20 per cent, with only Portugal amongst other members of the European Union spending less on social care.

If the thesis of this chapter that social care is functional is correct, the net result of recent changes should be dramatic. Indeed, if historical experience is a reliable guide, the failure to provide for adequate social care could well have explosive results not presently envisaged by policy makers. Against this conclusion there is currently little evidence of open dissent or public protest. Strike action has fallen to unprecedented levels. In fact, many observers tend to assume that Britain has come dramatically and abruptly to the end of its history of collective aggression and overt public protest. Such a view is just plausible enough to be taken seriously. Not only has the incidence of striking fallen away dramatically in the last twenty years of the twentieth century, but one can recognize that the traditional situation of conflictual industrial and social relations may have changed permanently. But it is not the case that the period since the early 1980s has no obvious historical precedent. With unemployment rising and strike frequency falling, the period 1920–30 is quite similar in many ways. As then, strike action would be extremely costly; as then, against the background of increasing relative poverty and the lack of welfare provision, the period has nevertheless featured the most bitter and bloody confrontations ever seen in British political history.

A scenario which envisages a rerun of the 1920s, however, in which there will be sudden and massive confrontations between capital and labour, is probably quite unlikely. It is not just that there are no longer any solidaristic working-class communities or that unions have been so weakened organizationally as to make effective action unlikely. At the same time there must be no underestimating the importance of the development of massive and seemingly permanent structural unemployment, which has been referred to by left (Mann, 1992) and right (Murray, 1990) as the emergence of 'the underclass'. No doubt it is the fear of losing one's job and landing up in the marginalized periphery of the economy, or out of it altogether, which concentrates the mind of potential strikers. However, perhaps the most important point to make is that rebellion, dissent and striking have always been undertaken by the *most disadvantaged* groups. The fact is that today people with ordinary jobs are not by any stretch of the imagination the disadvantaged. They are, in fact, people with much to lose. The most disadvantaged today are excluded from the economy in that they have no jobs at all. The most prevalent form of protest in the twentieth century – the strike – is thus not available to them. The underclass will progressively rediscover the effective forms of protest available from the traditional repertoire.

There is no reason to think that the age of collective public protest has ended, still less that there is no point in trying to preserve the welfare state. It can be argued that the virtual disappearance of the strike and the development of an economy and society in which it seems unlikely to be re-established as a viable form of political pressure are ominous facts and by no means an indication that the future will be free from conflict. Clearly, the opposite is true. In the view developed here, the traditional social settlement, in which state responsibility for full employment and social welfare was traded for domesticated industrial relations, has been abandoned. The rise of new forms of structural unemployment and greatly increased social need has occurred in the very years that state expenditure on welfare has been capped or reduced. This can hardly fail to alter patterns of protest fundamentally. It has changed both the kind of groups likely to engage in public protest and the means available to them. The emergence of the underclass as a greatly disadvantaged group with little to lose virtually guarantees that dissent, when it arrives, will be destructive and violent. In contrast to declining strike rates, the rising tide of lawlessness on public housing estates and recurrent unrest in the inner cities are events that are much more difficult to see in a positive light. These and other indications are clear signs of a return to collective violence. The riots in the inner cities in the 1980s and the destruction of prisons in more recent years suggest that the future will very likely be marked by sporadic, but sometimes spectacular, collective violence. From this view, it is the rise of the riot rather than the decline of the strike that is the key to the character of the present.

Of course, it is possible to dismiss rioting in the inner cities and the eruption of collective destructiveness and rebellion in the prisons as isolated instances of poor race relations, abrasive policing and/or ineffectual management. However, in contrast to this prevailing 'managerialist' orthodoxy about what is going wrong these sorts of events should be taken to give clear warning of the shape of things to come. They are an indication of the likely real costs of a withdrawing state and the effects of greatly reduced social care. As Britain approaches the meagre levels of social care which are deployed in the United States and adopts welfare policies which, as in the United States, leave pools of massive deprivation, we can expect the pattern of explosive conflict periodically seen in that country to appear in Britain too. When this occurs – which, on the balance of historical evidence, seems likely to be soon – don't care may be made to care.

Acknowledgments

The author would like to thank the following people for comments on the argument of this chapter at various points: Keith Soothill, Moira Peelo, Richard Hugman, John Scott, Colleen Thomas, Karen Legge and Paul Thompson.

Endnote

2.1. Hibbs also correlates state expenditure with left political representation in various countries and also finds strong correlations with three variables. This aspect of his work has given rise to considerable controversy and quite obviously raises lots of possibilities concerning the nature and direction of the causal relations between variables. I make no apology for avoiding discussion of such issues here.

References

Beer, S. 1965: *Modern British politics: a study of parties and pressure groups*. London: Faber.

Coates, D. 1994: *The question of UK decline: economy, state and society*. London: Harvester Wheatsheaf.

Cole, G.D.H. and Postgate, R. 1938: *The common people*. London: Methuen.

Cronin, J.E. 1979: *Industrial conflict in modern Britain*. London: Croom Helm.

Hibbs, D. 1978: On the political economy of longrun trends in strike activity, *British Journal of Political Science* 8(1), 135–75.

Hills, J. 1993: *The future of welfare: a guide to debate*. York: Joseph Rowntree Foundation.

Hobsbawm, E. 1968: *Labouring men*. London: Weidenfeld.

Hutton, W. 1995: *The state we are in*. London: Cape.

Jessop, R. 1979: Corporatism, parliamentariansm and democracy. In Schmitter, P.C. and Lembruch, G. (eds) *Trends towards capitalist intermediation*. London: Sage. 96–135.

Kemp, T. 1969: *Industrialisation in nineteenth century Europe*. London: Longman.

Kingdom, J. 1992: *No such thing as society*. Milton Keynes: Open University Press.

McBriar, A.M. 1962: *Fabian socialism and English politics*. Cambridge: Cambridge University Press.

Mann, K. 1992: *The making of an English 'underclass'*. Milton Keynes: Open University Press.

Marshall, T.H. 1950: *Citizenship and social class and other essays*. Cambridge: Cambridge University Press.

Marshall, T.H. 1977: *Class, citizenship and social development*. Chicago: University of Chicago Press.

Murray, C. 1990: *The emerging British underclass*. London: I.E.A. Health and Welfare Unit.

OECD 1994: *Employment outlook*. Geneva: OECD.

Sabine, G. 1951: *A history of political theory*. London: Harrap.

Shorter, E. and Tilly, C. 1974: *Strikes in France 1830–1968*. Cambridge: Cambridge University Press.

Smith, D. 1992: *Understanding the underclass*. London: Policy Studies Institute.

Thompson, E.P. 1968: *The making of the English working class*. Harmondsworth, Penguin Books.

Tilly, C. 1981: Introduction. In Tilly, A. and Tilly, C. (eds) *Class conflict and collective action*. London: Sage. 13–25.

Tilly, C., Tilly, L. and Tilly, R. 1974: *The rebellious century 1830–1930*. London: Dent.

Trebilcock, C. 1981: *The industrialisation of the continental powers, 1780–1914*. London: Longman.

Turner, B.S. 1986: *Citizenship and capitalism: the debate over reformism*. London: Allen and Unwin.

Turner, B.S. 1990: Outline of a theory of citizenship. *Sociology*. 24(2), 189–217.

Turner, B.S. 1993: Contemporary problems in the theory of citizenship. In Turner, B. (ed.), *Citizenship and social theory*. London: Sage. 1–18.

3

Community care: a unity of state and care? Some political and philosophical considerations

Graham B. McBeath and Stephen A. Webb

In this chapter we attempt to give some shape to the suspicion that community care is part of a broader political strategy effected by a government pursuing what has been called a 'New Right' agenda. For our purposes the term 'New Right' signifies a combination of neoliberal individualist morality, and the implications for economic policy of neoconservative overload theories of the welfare state. We focus particularly on this in the first section. In the second section we set out an argument which proposes some ways in which community care as a policy encompassing New Right thinking provides us with a bad copy of Hegel's civil society–state distinction (Hegel, 1942). Here we take issue with the social–policy and political science literature which suggests the distinction as it operates in New Right thought is drawn sharply. Rather, we point out that such a division, in terms of allocation of responsibility for welfare, is largely illusory.

The manufacturing of a new view of where state boundaries are to be drawn is itself part of a political strategy by which government insulates itself from being caught up in the old political conflicts surrounding resourcing of welfare. The neutralization of politics is attempted by allowing welfare provision to be developed via mechanisms of the market in the hope that the latter will be seen as a sphere analytically and substantively independent of the province of government.

Having made observations about the nature and character of community care as a facet of state practice and ideology from the standpoints of political sociology and political theory, we draw our chapter to a close by outlining a theory of care which takes account of the individual, this being an aspect of community care which is much stressed and which Hegel himself sees as the end point of civil society. In Hegel's interpretation of civic community, the generation of an understanding of the value of the 'other' and, ultimately, of society is the core issue. If we are to have a caring community, part of a view of care must seek to incorporate an account of relations between carer and the cared for. So in our theory of care, which transcends the questions of economic and political strategies to focus on how the moral ends of caring may be achieved, we make central the twin factors of the individual clients' subjective wishes and the structure of concern and understanding that ought to exist between client and provider.

As part of a theory of care we emphasize that, for a richer reading of the meaning of care, we need an account which develops the varying discursive contexts in which the meaning occurs. To this end, we have included consideration of the conditions of the social emergence of notions of care, recognizing that these are an interplay of forces such as religion, gender, family and morality. It will be seen that the subjective and objective dimension which we draw attention to in our analytical theory of care can be linked to the wider aspects of ethical rationalization at the level of the personal, and instrumental rationalization at the level of organization.

Community care: a New Right agenda?

Since the 1960s, 'community care' in various forms has been pursued in social policy and practice, but in the late 1980s it was given a more precise meaning embedded in beliefs and values – a discursive matrix – of individualism, familialism, voluntarism, managerialism and market accountability. To mention in succession so many 'isms' may suggest an infelicity of style, but more importantly it points towards there being some underlying structure of family resemblance or loose ideological affinity between the collocated terms. If one had to give an identification to this structure, one could call it 'neoliberalism'. Of course, there is never a perfect fit between a theoretically derived concept and some real-world example of it, but it is widely held in the literature that Conservative governments since 1979 have premised various of their welfare reforms upon ideas borrowed from the neoliberal thought of writers such as Hayek and Friedman as well as from the 'more conservative' analysis of governmental overload which came to prominence in political science around the mid-to-late 1970s (King, 1975). The latter more conservative economic arguments, of a necessary residualist strategy in public-sector provision of welfare in the face of escalating costs and therefore taxes, sat happily with the moral arguments of the neoliberals which favoured thrusting responsibility for an individual's welfare either on to that individual and his or her family or onto the voluntary and private sector on the grounds that individuals *qua* individuals have a primary duty of care for the self.

With regard to social and care services, the neoliberal moral and the conservative economic arguments do not of themselves insist on the presence of a competitive market in services. However, if some forms of competition between community care service providers emerge, it tends to drive down welfare costs to the state and thus satisfy the implication of the overload argument that the state must become less interventionist. The point here and above is to set out briefly the familiar pattern of ideological elements giving shape and purpose to community care today.

In policy terms the driving forces behind the late 1980s renegotiation of community care (the Audit Commission called it 'The community revolution') (1992)), have been the Griffiths Report (Griffiths DHSS, 1988) initiating debate, and the National Health Service and Community Care Act 1990 which put into law aspects and variants of the original Griffiths proposals.

The aim of community care is to maximize the opportunities of the user to receive best care correspondent with her or his ascertained needs while minimizing the need for institutionalization of the user. The latter is measured against the norm of persons living in ways they choose in their homes.

Just as there is a fit between the morality of neoliberalism and the economics of conservatism at the more general level, there is a clear fit between economics and morality at the level of community care. Essentially, the reduction of welfare dependence on impersonal state-funded structures such as residential homes implies both a return to the bosom of community and family and a transfer of welfare expenditure from high-cost institutional care to much lower cost social security benefits, social services and carer support.

To maximize or minimize in the ways I have just set out is to take as axioms of morality presumptions that subjectively speaking, the elderly, mentally ill and the disabled prefer to live outside of large-scale, autonomous institutions, and that objectively speaking, it is somehow better for these people to live in small-scale, familiar environments such as *their* road, *their* family, *their* house and so forth. This morality operates to some extent by default: that taking people out of institutions, or not putting people in them, must be good, because being in them is bad. A cynical rendering of the argument goes something like this:

1. community care endorses deinstitutionalization;
2. I am sceptical of Conservative governments, especially in matters of welfare;
3. however, institutions are terrible places, particularly mental hospitals;
4. Goffman says so;
5. there is a battery of psychological, psychiatric and physiological studies showing the mal-effects of institutionalization;
6. if I were in an institution I would hate it, be bored, regimented, etc.;
7. people should not be put into institutions;
8. we should take people out of institutions and put them into a caring community;

9. community care aims to do this, though we need lots of money to do it properly.

Obviously this is not a deductive argument, but it picks out the sort of reasons for community care offered by social workers heard by the present authors. The nature of such points is bound up with a rejection of statism and a preference for community arrangements. The latter is person-focused, the former institution-focused.

The running down of institutions because of starvation of funding to local government, and the expansion of private and voluntary elderly and mental homes, have found succour from a vivid if latent sense of the material and spiritual depravity of incarceration held by social workers and public alike. The popularization of studies of incarceration from Goffman (1968) and the writings of Garfinkel (1967), Laing (1960), Foucault (1965) and others has intellectually enhanced and in some way validated long-held public fears of the madhouse. Part of the problem of this delegitimization of large-scale institutionalized care is that it is arrived at through a crude reductionism. That is, that the critique of totalizing institutions encourages people to think that all public institutions of care and control are basically mausoleums to be feared. Thus if run-down local authority elderly homes can be interpreted as somehow like prisons, feelings about prisons can be imputed to elderly homes. However, fear of elder abuse and suspicions that private homes will cut costs and fail to offer a high level of care by using untrained, cheap staff means that there are doubts about the use of the private market in high-cost care as an alternative to state-run provision. Value bases have shifted such that the caring professions may positively prefer the community care strategy of leaving people in their own dwellings irrespective of need or client preferences and, in the first instance, without reference to costs.

What we want to suggest then is that social workers and others who would not always be a Conservative government's most wholehearted supporters, find the 1960s-type radicalism and imagery of decarceration deployed in community care attractive. This, combined with the dissemination of studies showing that people are better off in their own homes, as well as the persuasiveness of it being 'common sense', tends to preclude the thought that community care can be seen as an ideological manoeuvre which appeals to right as well as to left critics of 'the power structure'.

Part of the moral success of community care, then, derives from its bringing together of left radicalism and right libertarianism. This is grounded in its 'critique of total institutions', the obverse of which is anti-authoritarianism. The implicit political radicalism of community care recognized in the Audit Commission's use of the word 'revolution' is given a positive identity in focusing on user power, a bottom-up, demand-led view of services rather than a service-led top-down flow of local authority power.

Such political morality may prove popular with social workers, many of whom would like to see part of their role as being an advocate on behalf of the client 'against the system', even if the social workers are employed by a local authority.

The economic side of the community care proposals can be set firmly within a Conservative residualist agenda which focuses upon reduction of misallocation of public money. It places emphasis upon saving rather than spending and upon lower taxation, and, within the terms of the purchaser–provider structure, it places a focus upon market-style rationality encouraging competitive tenders to be sought outside of local authority services. This attempt to impose a change in the culture of social services away from in-house provision via administrative arrangements to an entrepreneurial role for the purchaser via the market was an implicit critique of bureaucracy. It would work on the notion of an antithesis between command economy and capitalism, between non-accountable bureaucracy and the discipline of the market which forces 'business' to be accountable to a rational agent's wish to obtain a good for the lowest negotiable price in the market place. Again we can link the economic with the moral in that bureaucracy links rhetorically to ideas of the impersonal, the uncaring, the inefficient and the unresponsive. Such a critique of bureaucracy which trades on public scepticism also entertains myths that 'things get done' when bureaucratic institutions are cut to the bone. This is allied to a gung-ho individualism presenting persons (entrepreneurs?) as better able to 'do it on their own' than rely on pettifogging administrators.

The point here is to identify elements legitimating community care strategy. In part the ideals of community care fit certain aspects of 'folk wisdom' about government failure as they do folk wisdom about total institutions and bureaucracy. These 'wisdoms' motivate forms of support for the contemporary idea of community care, as does the 'housekeeper' sensibility that one cannot endlessly spend on services without accountability to the taxpayer, which in turn justifies management control of budgets. Politically, the issues focus on the moral and financial appropriateness of government intervention and on the Nozickian type question of what the most extensive state should be (Nozick, 1974). For social policy, matters centre on a gradual shift away from the view that in Western democracies government has a positive duty to act as a comprehensive welfare state and to regulate private forms of provision. Now, it would seem, community care is a metonym for a reallocation of responsibilities of the modern state to a notionally separate part of human society, namely, what used to be called civil society. Maier has identified this problem as the *Changing boundaries of the political* (Maier, 1987). It is to the split between civil society and the state to which we now turn, arguing that Hegel's ideas of civil society are worth examining in the light of the interpretation we have given of community care.

Community care and civil society

The *locus classicus* for grasping the contours of civil society is that of Hegel's *Philosophy of right*. Along with it we have to consider his notions of the family and the state and how they relate to civil society. It is perhaps remarkable the extent to which one half of Hegel's account describes so well the social theoretical base of community care. As a result we would not seek to deny that we consider community care is civil society on the cheap!

In the literature, there is a basic distinction drawn between civil society and the state. Civil society is the public sphere and its means of regulation, and the state is the political sphere and its means of regulation. A person is a citizen, a sovereign individual and a subject of the state. The modern welfare state, however, did much to collapse the basic distinction by taking on responsibility for the maintenance of persons and their families via the politico-administrative structures of state. As Offe has pointed out, 'Political Sociologists . . . have seriously questioned the usefulness of the conventional dichotomy of "state" and "civil society". . . The delineation between "political" and "private" is becoming blurred' (Maier, 1987, p. 63).

Broad patterns of governmental intervention as the engine of dependency culture was seen, prior to 1979, as incontestably a morally necessary environment. Inevitably this made government the focus for citizen demands. Pressure-group politics was seen as an activity which occurred between legitimate organized interests and the appropriate department of state. Conflicting interest groups competed for the favour of the minister within the rule of law. Such was the nature of a simple liberal pluralism. The short-run cycle of electoral competition meant that political parties were forced to offer the public more and more welfare goods or at least agree to underwrite their means of delivery. Thus in the latter, where goods were delivered via the market, government was expected to regulate. An obvious case of this was the positive official reaction to greater regulation of the private housing market in the wake of 'Rachmanism'. (Rachmanism was a practice by slum landlords in the 1950s and 60s, of whom the most notorious was Peter Rachman, of evicting tenants in rent-controlled property by force).

The public ideology developed through the 1980s, with suspicion towards grand projects of the state (cf. Lyotard's *meta-recit*, 1984), having its most concrete manifestations in privatization of nationalized industries and some welfare services. Welfare being an issue closer to people's hearts than industry obliged government to be cautious. Some levels of oversight, regulation and public accountability had to be maintained. The legacy of Beveridge (long since abandoned by government but not by the public) was a myth politicians clung to for the purposes of public consumption while trying to develop means by which to escape the stranglehold of the myth. One such means was to articulate ideas which, though running counter to the comprehensive welfare state, would be acceptable to people. Ideas of independence, individualism, self-reliance, family support, non-interference in the private sphere, non-coercion and choice maximization were just the ticket. Between the two sets of ideas (state or market) was a trade-off point which was: the revitalization of community care.

Community care among other policies signals the retreat of the interventionist state and the forced opportunity for the reappearance of a doctrine of civil society. Hegel's division of civil society into various parts, and his general characterization of it, resembles the notion of the contours of what we choose to identify as the new civil society articulated by recent governments:

> In distinguishing civil from political society, Hegel recognised the emergence of a new social configuration: a separate, private social sphere, within which agents lived for themselves, without participating in political affairs. The heart of this new sphere was the modern market economy. Its form of life – the life of the bourgeois . . . was crucially shaped by the nature of capitalist economic relations (Hardimon, 1994, p. 190).

> Civil Society [is] an association of members as self-subsistent individuals in a universality which, because of their self-subsistence, is only abstract. Their association is brought about by their needs . . . and by an external organisation for attaining their particular and common interests (Hegel, 1942, section 157, p. 110).

Civil society becomes extrapolitical, with its own rationale and mechanisms of self-reproduction. It is a sphere in which one's interests are served by the dialectics of dependency between self and associations of which one is a member. 'It includes not only the modern market system, but also the legal and judicial system, a public authority responsible for social and economic regulation and the provision of welfare, and a system of voluntary associations.' (Hardimon, 1994, p. 191).

Of particular interest to us is the status given to public authorities and to voluntary associations. Under the public authority, private concerns such as one's welfare are recognized as rights which members of civil society hold as members of civil society against civil society. The voluntary associations or corporations are recognized as such by the state. They promote the interests of their members motivated in part because the organizers share or have a particular interest in the problems with which they deal. They offer a more personalized service than would the state. It is these corporations which for Hegel make people aware of the larger ends of society, and of their interdependent role in creating that society, or what he would see as a civic community. Public authority, too, promotes a sense of the civic community in providing essential services such as roads, welfare and education, which make for a reasonable society in which to live. In this way civil society reconciles individuality with society.

Membership of civil society comes from individuals nurtured in families. The family is the 'institutional complex within which people can develop and find recognition of . . . their emotional needs and traits' (Hardimon, 1994, p. 181). We act for another in our family out of love, not because of the other's rights or because of contract.

For Hegel the state is the conciliator between the various interests thrown up by modern society. Thus it is the point of mediation and transcendence of the particular for the sake of the universal.

In Hegel, the socio-political structure is the means by which the person is enhanced to fulfil his or her potential. This is a classic version of positive liberty. But it is questionable whether this is intended by the policy of community care. What we need to do now is to reinterpret our remarks on Hegel in the light of the current situation.

Community care as Hegelian civil society

Community care is an attempt to reallocate responsibilities from the public sector to Hegel's voluntary associations, to the market and to families. As *Caring for people* (DH, 1989, p. 24) puts it, 'The Government will expect local authorities to retain the ability to act as direct service providers, if other forms of service provision are unforthcoming or unsuitable'. The conditional 'if' indicates the shift in the balance from public to private arrangements. In the case of voluntary agencies, persons are not so much members of them as they are clients of voluntary providers of services contracted by the public sector. Local authorities prefer voluntary agencies to private companies because their primary aim is not profit but to work on behalf of the clients to provide good services of which they have expert knowledge (see Leat, 1993, p. 17). They are particularly involved in providing such and such a service which goes beyond the abstract interest in provision which private business and the state have. This resembles the reasoning of Hegel where corporations serve their members' interests by their organizers being particularly interested in the services themselves.

What needs to be stressed here is the government's multiple strategy of eviscerating dependency culture, improving allocative efficiency linked to budgetary control, developing a mixed economy of care, expecting families to take a greater role in caring for relatives and the depoliticization of social services expressed by administratively neutralizing the politics of welfare via an apparently simple contract between purchaser and provider. In the latter case, the central idea is for purchasers to become rational arbiters between needs claims and budgeting independently of political and moral rights. Given the aim to shift provision away from the politically sensitive public sector, the onus of responsibility will come finally to rest with independent providers who will be accountable to market discipline of losing the contract presuming alternative providers are available. Pressure-group politics is no longer at a premium as the territory and logic of accountability has changed to one of market rationality.

The point is that the discourse of community care and its operation can be located within a Hegelian conception of civil society or the family, in principle separable from that of the state. Governments set out the abstract system of rules which tend toward the constitution for a universal good, and civil society and the family articulate that at the level of the particular.

At the level of the carer and/or family the linkage with civil society is in terms of advice and support services to promote the well-being and thus the continuation of the work of the carer (see Audit Commission, 1992, p. 18). The idea of the family as being involved in caring because of the affective dimensions (for example Hegel's 'love for one's family') of relationships is drawn on. The worry to social services is that the carer will withdraw her or his labour. But guilt and shame are powerful incentives for relatives to become or continue to be carers. This in part happens because of neighbours' disapproval of 'putting granny away'. (Once again incarceration/decarceration imagery operates.)

The telos of the Hegelian system is the maximization of individual potential through the various structures of the civil society. This is a self-reflexive notion inasmuch as it is the expression of individual ends and interests. Community care has repeatedly stressed the idea of independence and choice maximization for those in need of care. The government notes this in *Caring for people*; the idea is to 'give people a greater individual say in how they live their lives and the services they need to help them to do so'. (DH, 1989, p. 4). The proposals as contained in various government documents are most unspecific about how individuals will have their say and in what way their wishes will be taken into account. The main focus for these are at the point of needs assessments, and though it is insisted that they should be needs led they will inevitably be forced to take account of budgetary concerns. As we have argued above, the basic assumption is that persons will want to stay in their own home or will wish to be returned to it as soon as possible. Almost *a priori* it is assumed that pursuing this course of action will be satisfying the goal of an individual.

The state is in a curious position; it is trying to run a welfare system as if it is independent of the state. Government stresses the need for provision initiatives to come from the independent sector which is in theory no part of government but is accountable to government because the public expect government to be responsible for welfare or at least its regulation. The neoliberal approach, of creating distinct spheres of responsibility which minimizes the work of government by handing that responsibility over to a much expanded civil society, which is in theory politically neutral, has had compromises forced on it. This has left little more than an illusion of a sharp civil society–state split, but it nonetheless should be seen that Conservative governments since 1979 have for ideological and financial reasons renegotiated the map of relations which existed between government, local authorities and the independent sector so that now the local authority, or more particularly social services, becomes Hegel's public authority that mediates between the other two on behalf of civil society.

We have given some exposition of how community care comes to stand for changes in the theory of the state in relation to welfare by suggesting that there are parallels to be drawn with a Hegelian view of civil society. But central to the project of Hegel and to neoliberals is the meaning of the individual. In what ways can the individual matter *qua* individual within a care system? Within budgetary constraints, satisfying the welfare needs and wants of the individual is problematic. This is perhaps where the values of neoliberalism clash with those of governmental overload theory which makes curtailing budgets a crucial feature. However, the imputation of choice and wishes into the agenda of community care gives a subjective turn to what it is to care for somebody. In the community care literature, needs-assessment procedures (which individuate needs and therefore persons), as we have noted, have little to say about the registering and uptake of wishes of the client.

In the next section we will explore what a theory of care should look like if it is to accommodate objective and subjective needs of the person to be cared for. We will argue that to develop care is to achieve a reciprocal understanding and thus validation of the care that is done. It is this understanding that consolidates a system of sympathy between carer and client and thereby moves beyond the rule-based prescriptions of government policy or impersonal services provided on the market or by social services. Hegel himself speaks of the corporation as like a second family because 'they are structured to care for their members' (Hardimon, 1994, p. 198). If through the organic connections between providers there is to be nurtured a relation of *gemeinschaft* rather than *gesellschaft* it could be pointed out that the former should rest on the development of personalized interaction and understanding.

Towards a theory of care

Care is an elusive concept. It is rarely addressed systematically in any literature, let alone in social work or health care literature. There are many books with 'care' in the title, but few, if any, discuss the concept theoretically. Thus much writing begs the question of the nature of care. For the most part analyses of care are about processes and policies which if carried out would be exemplary care practices in relation to a specific client-group. In other words, what care is, in terms of conceptual analysis, is left out of the account.

Within the 'caring' professions there is a presumption that practitioners practice care and that all their professional activities are strategies of care. The word 'care' tends to appear by default, independent of any consideration of what it may mean. It has been dispossessed of its moral power to call us to account for and reflect upon our practices – whether we are adhering to some root meaning of 'care' or not. It tends to function simply as a part of various phrases such as day care, social care and so forth. It has become a rather vague word that at best is used to capture a notion of improving someone's lot in life – raising their welfare function. In the 'caring' professions, care is a generic term for the sort of thing the professionals do. But it may be seen as generic in the sense of being a general term which is qualified by linking it to some more specific term such as elderly, child or health. Its use in the context of social work or nursing is taken for granted. It has a certain obviousness or 'appropriateness' because care, as some material practice, has always been understood to be the purpose of such professionals. 'Care' within the linguistic universe of agents of welfare makes no demands for any particular way of acting by those agents other than for acts specified by the real-world referents of types of care such as 'child care'.

However, if social services and health care professionals do not struggle with the meaning of the concept of care in their everyday practice, there will be few constraints on the way they do things for their clients. Criteria of good practice will tend to resolve around rather simplistic horizons of what are good ends for the client and what are efficient means of executing those good ends compatible with the law and with modes of practice set down by institutions and guidance manuals. It would seem to us that care is doing tasks in a way mindful of the objective and subjective reflected-upon interests of the person for whom the tasks are done. The primary sense of care, we suggest, is that found in the phrase 'taking care'. For the sort of thing we have in mind, we could point to care entailing that we do actions in such a way as to lessen the pain we are causing to someone by some treatment, given that we will cause *some* pain and it is the only treatment available. The person does not want any pain at all and may ask us not to continue to hurt them, but on reflection and consequent upon explanation from the carer the person realizes that some pain is an inevitable part of being cured which is what that person, the client, most wants. Here we are taking care (by minimizing pain but not compromising the treatment), and this is understood to be the case by the patient. What remains is a question of whether we are taking enough care subject to no greater harm being brought about or proscribed action being done by a 'more-care-taking' action. A less complicated example would be where one pulls an old lady away from an oncoming vehicle, hurting her in the pulling. Without this action, *ceteris paribus*, she would have been killed. Once she realizes this, it would be reasonable to claim that she would grant that one were taking care of her, though it did not seem to her to be the case initially.

The upshot of this preliminary analysis is that care related to the caring professions is a way of performing an action that is commonly understood as promoting the interests of a recipient by the recipient and the provider. This gives us a fairly formal definition within which is located the grounds for operationalization. By objective interests, as mentioned above, we mean the declared mutually agreed purpose(s) of intervention which in the normal course of things will take precedence over an epiphenomenal interest. Subjective interests are the ways performance or actions are done to satisfy the particular wants of the client/patient, where those wants arise during intervention. As a rule objective interests take precedence over subjective interests where they conflict. So, again taking an example from health: a patient has to be turned over every few hours, let us say from lying on the back to lying on the side. Subjectively, in the case of this patient the new position she or he has been placed in is uncomfortable because her or his legs are straight rather than drawn up. However, the patient is refused help to draw up her or his legs because it will inhibit blood flow or some such problem which in turn will inhibit the objective aims of the treatment.

To bring in a distinction between subjective and objective usually raises more problems than it solves, but it strikes us as necessary to use it to point up the relationship between the primary agreed purposes of intervention carried out according to typical, established or prescribed ways of doing an action, and the ways of doing this desired by the recipient. It must be acknowledged that objectivity is often deepened by goals being determined by a metagoal which only the most extreme conditions of say, a patient, can override. For instance, all hospital treatment starts from a premise of intervention aiming at not accelerating death and in most circumstances aiming at the prolongation of life. No matter how bad a patient's condition, euthanasia is rarely the first option to be considered. Not to think of euthanasia or not letting someone die is not merely a moral inhibition but a disposition inculcated through training, institutionalized values and routine practices which automate responses to situations without reference to rules and the evaluation of their validity.

There are, then, backstops or higher-order rules and goals by which lower-order, concrete interventions are circumscribed. The latter are, themselves, institutionalized, routinized or prescribed – what we might call 'established'. These constitute one side of the face-to-face taking-care process and which may be varied, subject to higher order objectively determined constraints, as a result of the subjective wants of the patient (or the carer).

Our concept of care is not a *a priori* but rather a theoretical account shaped by empirical considerations. Our notion of objective serves to recognize the objectivizing processes through which treatments and interventions pass. We could of course simply reduce our account to one of utility of interventions in terms of causing more or less harm and do away with the objective–subjective distinction. But this would discount the presence of social processes and interactions and thereby of sociological observation which in turn would reduce the thickness of definition we are seeking to achieve.

To round off our thoughts about the nature of care, we should briefly look at other uses of the term. In the phrase 'I really care for you', care is disconnected from qualifying an action. Here it is a statement of openness toward concern for someone without specification of criteria of caring. It is a mental disposition. The phrase 'I don't really care for him' in its most colloquial form is again a mental disposition indicating a point along a continuum running between disinterest and not liking someone. By varying the intonation we can convey that we mean that we are not a primary carer of someone, as in '*I* don't really care for him . . . someone else does'. One last phrase we might pay attention to is that of 'having a duty of care'. That is warrantably to look after and imposes an obligation to ensure that within one's jurisdiction, in terms of time or space, no (further) harm visits a person or group of persons. In respect of health and social services this is preventive rather than facilitative. As such it does not correspond with our definition of care above. It is not primarily concerned with ways of doing, nor with goals of positively caring for, but rather with ensuring that someone does not make themselves worse off. It is an inverted form of pareto optimality.

'Care' discourse

Our analytical distinction between the subjective and the objective dimensions of the concept of care can, of course, be translated into a more straightforward sociological reading of the 'discourse of care' as it comes to be deployed as a legitimating device for the caring professions. Such a reading, drawing on the pioneering work of Weber (1947), Sombart (1967) and the critical theorists (Horkheimer, 1972) would more directly emphasize the historical and social construction of care as an ideological tool which performs a crucial strategical function for both the control of the recipients of care and the legitimation of professional power. In this respect we can draw attention to the rationalizing processes of social life within Western societies and the productive canalizing of these processes within institutional and professional contexts. Here we can trace the ways in which the contemporary usage of concept of care is dialectically constituted by specific discursive arrangements, which at a subjective level are founded on an ethical rationalization of personal life and which at an objective level derive from an instrumental rationalization of organizational life. Put simply, current usages of the concept of care are formed as an effect of the strategic conjunction of these two dimensions of social rationalization which produce particular ways of thinking about personhood, ethical interpersonal relations and moral communities. Thus the contemporary preoccupation with and usage of the concept of care has a specific history.

The emergence of 'care' can be traced to changes in self-understandings which were themselves connected to a wide range of religious, economic, moral, sexual and familial discourses. Taylor (1989), has convincingly shown that 'the Enlightenment and Romanticism with its accompanying expressive conception of mankind, have made us what we are. . . . Certain moral ideas emerge from this crucial period which still form the moral horizon of our outlook. One thing the Enlightenment has bequeathed us is a moral imperative to reduce suffering. . . . Another major idea we have seen developing is that of the free, self-determining subject' (pp. 393–5). In other words, it is likely that the concept of care would not have emerged either an institutionalized professional practice or a measure of the moral veracity of interpersonal relations without a corresponding change in the definitions of subjectivity and liberal morality. In this respect, other obvious examples of the changing nature of caring relationships include the advent of philanthropic and charitable work; new child-rearing practices which developed from the eighteenth century onwards; the demarcation and defence of privacy, and public concern to maintain it; the cultivation and display of sentiment in romantic affairs; gender divisions in the domestic sphere; and increasing state intervention in family life (see Meyer, 1983; Sombart, 1967). Foucault (1986) in the *Care of the self* places this emerging conception of an ethical self much further back in ancient Greek culture and points to three general processes in the historical formulation of the care for personhood:

- the individualistic attitude, characterized by the absolute value attributed to the individual in his or her singularity, and by the degrees of independence conceded to him or her via the group to which he or she belongs and the institutions to which he or she is answerable;
- the positive valuation of private life, that is, the importance granted to family relationships, to the forms of domestic activity and to the domain of patrimonial interests;
- the intensity of the relations of self, that is, of the forms in which one is called upon to take oneself as an object of knowledge and a field of action so as to transform, correct and purify oneself and find salvation.

He goes on to show how this 'cultivation of self', which is so highly prized in the modern training of members of the caring professions, is dominated by the principle that one must 'take care of oneself' (p. 43). These processes, for Foucault, give rise to new institutional practices and modes of knowledge, which, we would argue, culminate in the modern caring profession, its values, practices and knowledge base.

We can summarize this section by noting that these discourses contribute to a developing set of practical arrangements which increasingly invoke the concept of care and either demarcate or join the relationships between privatized individuals, gender differences, emerging welfare state institutions and changing economic markets. These relations must not be confused with a unidirectional causal structure. It is just as important to note the way in which the formulation of concepts of care in the caring professions smoothes the way for the extension of the concept in economic and market relations as it is to point to the increased penetration of market ideology within the caring professions themselves, and how economic practices made it more natural for caring professionals to see themselves as reflecting these practices. The causal arrow runs in both directions between the discourse and the practice of care.

Conclusions

In this chapter, we have reviewed some of the developments in community care by setting them against the backdrop of theories of the state and legitimation of the strategies by which such theories become acceptable. Community care is an instructive example of how a significant shift in the relation between state and people is negotiated. We also indicated how this relation is situated within broader social and historical processes which convey various discursive and power-laden regimes of professional practice.

It is our view that community care has played fast and loose with the notion of community, the government knowing that the word 'community' has positive connotations. The policy to a great extent has been focused on attempts to control welfare budgets. We sought to explore the policy in the context of the political economy of what has been called the 'New Right' and of its social and moral aims. Perhaps our largest context has been the debate still going on which is concerned with the limits of state identity and action. The renegotiation of the boundaries of the state is not a debate between the modern and the postmodern state but rather between one conception of the modern state and another. Elsewhere we have argued that if fragmentation of welfare was occurring it was a controlled fragmentation (McBeath and Webb, 1991). That is, provision of social services was being administered under a stricter division of labour than previously. What we did not stress, then, was that this process tended to lift the burden of accountability from the state and change its form. We hope we have successfully pointed this out here.

Our section titled 'Towards a theory of care' was a response to what we saw as the need for examining the nature of care by providing an account which addressed itself to the hope for care that recognized the personal and subjective dimension of need in the face of a more cynical analysis of the motivations of the current care systems. Here the importance of care should lie with the individual recipient, thus at least fulfilling more nearly one aspect of a Hegelian civil society of which, we argued, community care offered us a bad copy. Finally, we noted the importance of situating contemporary usages and practices of care within specific historical and social contexts through which a discourse of care has emerged in modern Western societies. This we suggested would enable practitioners and researchers to understand better the relations of power and ideological constructs which are at work in the ordinary and everyday usages of the term 'care'.

Acknowledgements

The authors would like to thank Pamela Abbott and Kevin Pettican for their comments.

References

Audit Commission 1992: *The community revolution.* London: HMSO.
DH 1989: *Caring for people.* Department of Health. London: HMSO.
Foucault, M. 1965: *Madness and civilisation.* London: Tavistock Publications.
Foucault, M. 1986: *Care of the self.* Middlesex: Penguin.
Garfinkel, H. 1967: *Studies in ethnomethodology.* New Jersey: Prentice Hall.
Goffman, E. 1968: *Asylums.* Middlesex: Penguin.
Griffiths, Roy/DHSS 1988: *Community care-agenda for action: a report to the Secretary of State for Social Services.* London: HMSO.
Hardimon, M. 1994: *Hegel's social philosophy.* Cambridge: Cambridge University Press.
Hegel, G.W.F. 1942: *Philosophy of right*, Knox, (trans.) Oxford: Oxford University Press.
Horkheimer, M. 1972: *Critical theory.* New York: Continuum.
King, A. 1975: Overload: problems of governing in the 1970's, *Political Studies* **23**.
Laing, R.D. 1960: *The divided self.* Middlesex: Penguin.
Leat, D. 1993: *The development of community care by the independent sector.* London: Policy Studies Institute.
Lyotard, J.F. 1984: *The postmodern condition.* Manchester: Manchester University Press.
Maier, C.S. 1987: *Changing boundaries of the political.* Cambridge: Cambridge University Press.
McBeath, G.B. and Webb, S.A. 1991: Social work, modernity and postmodernity. *Sociological Review* **39**(4), pp. 745–62.
Meyer, P. 1983: *The child and the state: the intervention of the state in family life.* Cambridge: Cambridge University Press.
National Health Service and Community Care Act 1990: *Public general acts – Elizabeth II* chapter 19. London: The Stationery Office.
Nozick, R. 1974: *Anarchy, state and utopia.* Oxford: Blackwell.
Sombart, W. 1967: *Luxury and capitalism.* Ann Arbour, MI: University of Michigan Press.
Street-Porter, J. 1981: *Scandal.* London: Penguin.
Taylor, C. 1989: *Sources of the self: the making of the modern identity* Cambridge: Cambridge University Press.
Weber, M. 1947: *The theory of social and economic organisation.* Glencoe IL: Free Press.

Part 2: Developments in formal care services

Editors' introduction

For better or worse, there have been major changes in formal care services in many countries over the past decade. In Britain, the implementation of the National Health Service and Community Care Act 1990 incorporated reform in health and social services provision, based on the creation of a competitive market. As there was no precedent for such a system within the UK and experience abroad was also limited the scale of the experiment has been described as quite remarkable.

The Act altered traditional power bases in a significant way: the most crucial shift in setting up the internal health market in Britain is the requirement that all district health authorities should divide themselves into purchasers and providers. So, for example, district health authorities are just one kind of purchaser, and the Act also provided for groups of general practitioners (GPs), that is, primary health care physicians, to become fundholders. Hence, the GPs involved are allocated budgets out of the funding that would previously have gone to health authorities. While the GP fundholding scheme only began on a small scale, there were some early signs that it may prove effective in improving care standards as GPs 'shop around' in order to get better services for their patients (Harrison, 1992, p. 12). However, it could eventually prove to be the case that the extra administration involved may offset these possible benefits and some unintended consequences may follow. The organizational and financial reforms contained in the 1990 Act may be modified as elections come and go. However, it seems that the introduction of policies for achieving better health based on prevention rather than treatment are rather more fundamental realignments.

In fact, most of the discussions in the UK have focused upon the effect of these shifts in interprofessional relations, especially on the medical profession and their relationship with the new cadre of managers (for example, Walby *et al.*, 1994). In Chapter 4, in contrast, Quinney, Pearson and Pursey describe conceptualizations of 'care' within primary health care nursing: they point to how these nurses' conceptualizations of care can be seen to lie along a continuum of models of health, from the highly biomedicalized model at one end to a psychosocial environmental model at the other. More importantly, they identify how the nurses' situation is dynamic rather than static. So where nurses figure on this continuum depends to a large extent on what are varying organizational contexts and circumstances, which lend themselves to different approaches to 'care'. In fact, while nurses themselves rarely recognize the relevance of the wider socio-political context, it is argued that this has been crucial in influencing primary health care nurses' practice and relations with clients and other professionals. Quinney, Pearson and Pursey conclude by identifying a possible paradox. In beginning to understand the structures and culture of the internal National Health Service market, they suggest that 'the apparently relentless and mechanistic "logic" of the internal market will thwart one its avowed aims: of affording people greater choice and ensuring services which better meet their needs' (p. 70). This may be a message which the rest of the world may also need to consider in terms of evaluating the experiments in health and social care carried out in Britain in the 1990s.

In Chapter 5, using the Australian allied health professions as a case study, Boyce identifies a fundamental change which has been occurring as part and parcel of 'reforms' of the health sector. So, while professions report both positive and negative effects on their power, autonomy and control over the context of care, it is organizational and managerial factors – that is, factors outside the clinical care domain – which are increasingly setting the agenda. In her case study, Boyce traces the emergence of an 'allied health movement' at national, state and organizational levels She argues that the cultural change achieved in such new organizational approaches can, in turn, be a catalyst which drives changes at the national and state levels. While it may be premature to suggest the imminent arrival for the allied health professions of a new and liberating relationship with medicine, there seems little doubt that interprofessional relations are currently in flux (Soothill *et al.* 1995) and that there are similarities in developments among the Australian, Canadian and British therapy professions.

References

Harrison, A. (ed.) 1992: *Health care UK 1991*. London: King's Fund Institute.

National Health Service and Community Care Act 1990: *Public general acts – Elizabeth II* chapter 19. London: The Stationery Office.

Soothill, K., Mackay, L. and Webb, C. (eds) 1995: *Interprofessional relations in health care*. London: Edward Arnold.

Walby, S., Greenwell, J., Mackay, L. and Soothill, K. 1994: *Medicine and nursing: professions in a changing health service*. London: Sage.

4

'Care' in primary health care nursing

Deborah Quinney, Maggie Pearson and Ann Pursey

Introduction

The aim of this chapter is to describe conceptualizations of 'care' within primary health care (PHC) nursing[4.1] and to consider critically the factors which have shaped them. Drawing on evidence from a recent empirical study of PHC nursing in the north of England, we argue that the nature of 'care' as practised by PHC nurses'[4.2] is varied and is shaped by the organizational context in which it is practised, which in turn reflects the socio-political framework within which health care is delivered in the UK. In particular, we will argue that PHC nurses' conceptualizations of care can be seen to lie along a continuum of models of health: from the highly biomedicalized model at one end to a psychosocial environmental model at the other. Whilst individual nurses displayed a general tendency towards one end of the continuum or the other, in reality they were not always 'fixed' in one position. Rather, their location changed to some extent in different organizational contexts and circumstances which lend themselves to different approaches to 'care'.

Nurses themselves rarely conceptualize their care with individual clients with reference to the wider socio-political context, but we argue that the dominant ideology of the market, which has underpinned the reform of health care organization and provision in the UK in the 1990s (Ferlie, 1994) has influenced PHC nurses' practice and relations with clients and other professionals. By considering PHC nurses' differing conceptualizations of care, we attempt to explain why some nurses feel (and arguably are) under threat, whilst others are thriving in the new market economy (Hiscock and Pearson, 1996).

The chapter is structured as follows: first, we discuss key recent developments in UK health policy which have had a major impact on the organization and nature of PHC nursing and on its importance in the delivery of health care. We then consider the current organization of PHC nursing in the UK and the effect of recent policy developments before going on to discuss the findings of a qualitative study in the north of England of PHC nurses' 'care' in practice. Finally, we consider the implications of these findings for our understanding of PHC nurses' concepts of care.

Key developments in UK health policy

Two sets of recent developments in UK health policy have had specific implications for the organization and practice of PHC nursing: first, the introduction of market mechanisms, and, second, the increasing prominence of primary health care within the National Health Service (NHS) as a whole.

The introduction of market mechanisms

Since 1989 the NHS has been undergoing the most radical reform since its inception in 1948. In common with other Western nations, an internal health care quasi-market has been established which, it was assumed, would inevitably and uniquely improve efficiency (DH, 1989a; Ferlie, 1994). Health care is now 'purchased' from health care providers, some of whom are in direct competition with each other, by local health authorities or by 'fundholding' general practitioners (GPs) who hold specific funds for the purchase of a specific list of procedures (DH, 1989a, 1994; NHSME, 1992). Health services for the local populations of health districts or specific general practices are therefore defined in contracts with health care providers which stipulate the volume, nature, cost (and quality) of specific services, including 'community nursing',[13] which GP fundholders have been able to purchase directly since 1993 (NHSME, 1992).

The introduction of market mechanisms and contracting processes has brought with it specific management information requirements to support the 'measurement' and monitoring of service activity (Bennet and Ferlie, 1994; Freemantle et al., 1993; Ham, 1992). In general medical practice, which was established within the NHS in 1948 on the basis of contracts with independent medical practitioners for the provision of general medical services, a new contract negotiated simultaneously with the introduction of market principles included measurable targets for practice population coverage in preventive services such as cervical screening and immunizations (DH, 1989b). With concerns about value for money driving the market reforms, contracting is developing from an initial concern with input costs and service activity to a more sophisticated focus on clinical process and outcomes which can be measured and monitored (Flynn et al., 1995). Health care purchasers and providers are being encouraged to withdraw from the NHS some clinical procedures which have been shown to have no 'evidence-base' or to be of questionable utility and outcome (DH, 1993). Whilst this general shift towards a scientific basis for clinical interventions is laudable, critics and health care practitioners argue that this rational–technical goal with its focus on measurable activity and tasks is being pursued at the expense of more holistic, supportive and 'softer' aspects of health and health care which may not be so tangible or easily quantifiable (Hiscock and Pearson, 1996; Wilkinson, 1995).

The increasing prominence of primary health care

Primary health care has become increasingly significant in the provision of health care in the UK since the late 1980s as health policy has purposefully shifted the balance of care from hospitals and other institutions to primary and community care settings (DH, 1989c; DHSS, 1987). In addition, a new contract for general medical practitioners' services, introduced in 1990, included new incentives to expand preventive health care and disease management services in general practice (DH, 1989b), and there has been a generally increasing emphasis in health policy and practice on health promotion (DH, 1992). In promoting and strengthening primary care, national and local health policy has encouraged the development of primary health care teams, which are seen as playing a key role in the further development of the NHS to being more 'primary-care-led' in both the commissioning and the provision of health care (DH, 1994). Thus, whether fundholding or not, general medical practice is intended to become a focal point for strategy, planning and purchasing of health services in addition to continuing its traditional role in providing primary health care for patients.

Primary health care nursing in the UK

PHC nursing in the UK can be defined as the work undertaken by those nurses working in the public-sector NHS and who work outside hospitals or nursing homes. Such primary health care services often have general medical practice (hereafter referred to as 'general practice') as their organizational focus and may be delivered in a range of settings, including: people's own homes; community-based health clinics; and GPs' own surgery premises. These nurses' activities are generally focused on individuals or groups within a local, geographically defined population, which is usually the population registered with a specific general practice.[44]

PHC nursing is complex and varied, comprising, on the one hand, a range of nursing services provided by community health service provider organizations who employ 'community nurses', and, on the other, practice nurses employed directly by GPs. Until April 1996 community nursing and practice nursing were organized under the auspices of separate yet complementary health authorities usually covering the same geographical area: district health authorities (DHAs) which, like GP fundholders, purchased community health services; and family health services authorities

(FHSAs), under whose auspices practice nurses were employed by GPs. The two types of authorities united in April 1996, but differences in the employment arrangements for community nurses and practice nurses persist. Whereas community nurses are employed by community health service providers, which in turn have contracts for services with health authorities and GP fundholders, practice nurses are employed directly by GPs, in whose primary health care teams they work, alongside community nurses. We will argue that PHC nurses' positions in the health care market, as reflected in their different employment arrangements and contractual contexts, are, and have been, crucial factors shaping the nature of their practice.

Primary health care nursing teams?

Nurses working in primary health care settings are clearly a heterogeneous group who were previously considered as separate disciplines and subdisciplines with their own specific bodies of knowledge and practice. Indeed, in a major review of community nursing services (excluding practice nursing) 10 years ago, Cumberledge described them as 'hemmed inside' their own professional disciplines (DH, 1986). Nevertheless, the generic term 'primary health care nurses' is increasingly used in policy documents within the NHS as a single term including 'practice nurses' and 'community nurses', which emphasizes the officially perceived scope for them to work in 'primary health care teams' (NHSME, 1993). Such teams had often previously been understood to include only GPs and their own practice nurses. Despite their organizational and contractual differences and professional subspecialties, practice nurses and community nurses are, as 'PHC nurses', increasingly expected to collaborate and to be substitutes for each other as part of an intentional strategy to overcome fragmentation, duplication, gaps and overlaps in PHC nursing.

The focus of this chapter

This chapter focuses on three principal types of PHC nurses, each of which is categorized as generalist and which together compose over 85 per cent of the PHC nursing workforce: practice nurses, health visitors and district nurses. Of the 50 000 whole time equivalent nurses working in primary health care in England and Wales, almost two fifths are district nurses, approximately a quarter are health visitors and just over a fifth are practice nurses employed by GPs (Hirst et al., 1995). The number of practice nurses has trebled since 1988, in contrast to district nurses and health visitors whose numbers have remained stable, despite the higher profile of primary health care (DH, 1995; Hirst et al., 1995). Other nurses make an important contribution to primary health care, including community psychiatric nurses, community paediatric nurses and nurses working with people with learning disabilities, but we do not include them here because our study focused specifically on the numerically most prominent group of 'generalist' nurses working with older people and with mothers with young children.[45]

Health visitors work in preventive health care, surveillance and health promotion, and hold a generic title which implies that they work across a total population. In reality, most work principally with families with young children (Luker and Orr, 1992). The specialist branch of health visiting for older people was established in part as a response to the generic health visitors' concentration on work with young families (BSG/HVA, 1986) and in response to growing concerns about the needs of older people living at home (DHSS, 1981). These health visitors work predominantly with older people who are deemed to be 'in need' (often those with chronic illnesses and/or requiring monitoring) but who do not require the skills or attention of a district nurse. Historically, health visiting has perceived itself to be more autonomous than other branches of nursing (de la Cuesta, 1992).

District nurses tend to work with a wide range of the population, although 80 per cent of patients on their caseload are over 65 years of age (Badger *et al.*, 1989). Their work is determined largely by demand for specific types of nursing intervention within the home setting, which may be specifically ordered by a GP (for example, taking blood for tests; dressing a wound) or a hospital at the time of discharge (for example, dressing a wound; insulin injections). The district nurse may decide upon the specific interventions required after assessing a patient's needs, again at the request of a GP or a hospital.

The nature of practice nurses' work is determined largely by their GP employers, and much of their activities are delegated tasks which are required in order for those GPs to fulfil their contracts to provide general medical care for a registered list of patients (DH, 1989b; Pursey, 1992).

In the remainder of this chapter, we explore similarities and differences in the practice of these three principal types of PHC nurses, drawing upon data from a recent empirical study of PHC nursing in one health district in the north of England (Quinney and Pearson, 1996). The study was funded by the Department of Health specifically to identify and explore the impact of the health policies outlined above on PHC nurses' practice. A total of 46 periods of observation and 17 interviews were undertaken with 27 PHC nurses working with four general practice populations. The sample of nurses comprised 11 practice nurses, employed directly by general practitioners; 10 district nurses (including 4 unqualified auxiliary nurses); and 6 health visitors, of whom 4 worked principally with families with young children, and 2 worked with older people. The four general practices were selected to reflect the wide range of socio-economic conditions within the district and differences in GP fundholding status in the district. Specifically, the study sought to identify and explore PHC nurses' relationships and interactions with clients and colleagues, their own descriptions of their roles and responsibilities and the content and nature of their practice.

The qualitative methodology and in-depth observations generated a complex and rich picture of nurses' interactions with their clients and enabled insights into the implicit and explicit concepts and principles underpinning their practice. This methodology also revealed the more intangible dimensions of nursing practice which are not easily quantified or reflected in questionnaire surveys, management information systems or current service contract performance indicators. Here, we summarize the empirical findings, which are reported more fully elsewhere (Quinney and Pearson 1996), and draw upon them to explore meanings of 'care' in PHC nursing practice.

Different approaches to 'care' in nursing practice

Our research in the north of England identified differences in each group of PHC nurses' practice which reflected variations in the meanings of nursing 'care'. These differences were manifest in nurses' degree of professional autonomy, including responsibility for, and decision making about, treatments and the care of clients;[16] the extent to which their practice was delegated by and subsidiary to that of other PHC professionals, in collaboration with them; and the degree to which their practice was reactive to clients' concerns or proactive, imposing an agenda upon them.

Within the variations of the four groups of nurses' practice, two distinct approaches were observed: on the one hand, a task-orientated, functional approach, in which nursing 'care' was fragmented into its component parts; and, on the other, a person-orientated, supportive approach, in which the component parts of nursing 'care' were integrated within an holistic framework. These distinct approaches are 'idealized types' in the sense that they sit at opposite ends of a continuum of conceptualizations of care as manifest in nursing practice, but they are not in fact mutually exclusive. Indeed, individual nurses were observed to combine elements of both or, as in the case of some district nurses, to have a very task-orientated approach to the initial contact with a household, which developed over time, during repeated contacts, into a more 'holistic' approach as the nurse became more familiar with the client and his or her family.

A number of factors were found to shape the content and nature of a PHC nurse's practice and 'care', most notably organizational management requirements, employment arrangements, contractual obligations to achieve targets and statutory responsibilities, such as a health visitor's duties in respect of child protection. Where organizational and contractual requirements were a key influence on a nurse's practice, the limits of her own responsibilities were clearly demarcated.[17] Where the nurse's practice was less closely stipulated in contracts or verbal agreements she was observed to have more personal influence on the nature of the care she provided and was more able to respond to her client's own concerns.

Nursing as 'doing' functional tasks

In the functional approach to PHC nursing practice, an interaction between a client and nurse focuses largely on a task or set of tasks which need to be 'done', such as a dressing, an injection, a strip wash, weighing babies or child development checks. The nurse's role and functions are described in terms of what they concretely 'do' for people. As one practice nurse described:

> I mainly do a mixed bag of all sorts: take bloods; blood pressure checks; new patient checks; smears; vaccinations for holidays; dressings; ear syringing; most things really.

Such 'tasks' often need only one client–nurse contact, in which the purpose of the interaction is clearly demarcated. This approach is reminiscent of the task-orientated approach to nursing still found in some hospitals (Reed, 1984; Waters, 1991), in which nurses fragment the body (Turner, 1992) into a series of physical needs to be met. Interactions between different nurses and a single patient are episodic and discontinuous, the task-orientated interaction with the client being a completed episode in itself. Indeed, in primary care, a client may see different nurses in successive contacts, as in baby clinics, wound clinics or general practice nurse clinics. In these strictly bounded interactions, which focus on a limited, physical component of a client's 'health', there is little scope for the feeling or emotional aspects of care, although some clients in our study were observed to comment that, in undergoing these screening activities, they felt 'cared for'. This approach reflects a narrowly biomedical model of health, most clearly evident in monitoring and surveillance health checks and clinics undertaken principally by practice nurses but also by health visitors in specific clinical settings. District nurses and health visitors for older people were rarely observed to practice nursing 'care' in this way, but it must be emphasized here that they were not observed to undertake any clinics as such. In some districts, district nurses may run 'specialist' clinics, such as for leg ulcers.

In general practice, most screening activities performed by practice nurses are perceived to be a means of identifying problems which can then be referred on to the GP or another health care professional. The annual health check for people aged over 75 years, which is a requirement of the GP contract typically fulfilled by practice nurses who may be specifically appointed for this purpose (DH, 1989b; Harris, 1992; Nocon, 1992), is a 'one-off' event which is repeated annually. It involves an assessment of a person's health in order to identify the unmet needs of older people within a general practice population. The checks commonly use a predetermined checklist which principally comprise physiological parameters (blood pressure; urine content) and biological functions (continence; appetite; hearing) to assess a person's 'health'. Any deviations from physiological or biological norms would be followed up by further checks and by diagnostic tests and examination by the GP if necessary. We observed that, when broader health or social care problems were identified during these checks, they were rarely followed up by the nurse herself. Rather, the older person was advised about the action to take himself or herself. For example, when a client was identified as probably being clinically depressed that client was advised to make an appointment to see the doctor. There was no follow up by the nurse herself, and the next contact between the nurse and client would be scheduled for the annual check the following year. This confirms the findings of another recent study of annual health checks (Pursey, 1992).

The discontinuity of contact was both observed and reported to affect potentially the nurse–client relationship. In one case, a practice nurse revisiting an older woman for the annual check was greeted with considerable anger because the identification during the previous year's check of her 'need' for a bath rail, which had been referred on to social services, had not resulted in any action. The older woman made it clear that she felt the annual check (and, by strong inference, the nurse herself) was worthless. Another practice nurse, whose work was divided between doing the annual checks at one surgery and doing the checks and a clinic session at another, valued the scope in the second setting to 'bring patients in' to follow up problems identified during the check. She clearly regretted the impossibility of this at the surgery where she only undertook the checks in people's own homes.

The task to be 'done' similarly dominated some PHC nurses' clinic activities classed, for the purposes of GPs' reimbursement under the 1990 GP contract, as health promotion or, more recently, as disease management (DH, 1989b). Indeed, practice nurses' 'care' often comprised no more or less than the clearly defined task itself. The key objective for practice nurses in such clinics was to influence and encourage change in clients' lifestyles, including diet, exercise, smoking, alcohol consumption and other behaviours identified as risk factors for certain diseases. Advice and information was observed to be given frequently by nurses about particular diseases which were the focus of the clinic, such as coronary heart disease, diabetes or asthma, but clients were rarely encouraged, or observed, to discuss or challenge it. Rather, they appeared to accept what they were told as expert knowledge, even though the relevance of the advice and information to their own situation may be questionable. Although the concept of client participation is regarded as fundamental in effective health promotion, where issues were raised by clients which were not related to the nurse's own task-orientated agenda they were rarely followed through, unless it was a request for specific information.

Four aspects of this approach to nursing 'care' are worth noting here. First, the task-specific activities are characteristically undertaken by PHC nurses as 'subsidiary' carers, in support of, and in response to, other primary and secondary care professionals' practice. Their practice and nursing 'care' can be seen as working towards an agenda set externally to their interaction with a client. For example, some treatments and monitoring regimes, such as for diabetes or asthma, were 'prescribed' by secondary care providers, and clients were referred back to secondary care when necessary. Second, these interactions were more likely to take place in the health centre or clinic, where sessions are strictly time tabled and where the client may have pressing needs which require practical advice and assistance.

Third, this task-orientated practice is tangible and can be measured relatively easily in 'process' terms of task completion, such as the number of health checks done, the number of hypertensions detected, the number of clinic attendances and so on. It lends itself more easily to simple 'outcome' measurement than other, 'softer', types of nursing care, hence appealing to the drive within the NHS for clear specification of function and measurement of activity. In fact, it is the process and what the nurse has done or completed which is measured rather than the outcome or effectiveness of the task or any long-term health gain (Flynn *et al.*, 1995). This concern with counting tasks is actively encouraged by 'items of service' payments and financial incentives for the achievement of population targets for GP screening services (DH, 1989b). The effectiveness of the tasks and the nurses' practice is rarely disputed. Practice nurses' activities in particular were undertaken in order to meet the needs of the service, as set out in their GP employer's contractual obligations to offer health checks for people aged over 75 years, and to meet population targets for 'health promotion' screening for disease risk factors, infant vaccinations, child development checks and cervical screening. Other PHC nurses employed by community health care providers with health authority and GP fundholders contracts for services were also involved in such task-specific activities, as part of their employer's contractual obligations to contribute towards the achievement of those targets. In this and another, simultaneous, study in two other health districts (Hiscock and Pearson, 1996), health visitors working within service contracts with GP fundholders reported that they were being required to give this strictly bounded and easily measurable task-orientated activity precedence over more supportive, holistic approaches to working with families with young children. The activities of nurses using this approach are generally delegated or prescribed by the GP who, in the case of the practice nurse, is their employer (Pursey, 1992), or in the case of GP fundholders and community nurses, their 'quasi-employer' (Hiscock and Pearson, 1996). Indeed, for some groups of patients (for example, those with asthma or heart disease), GPs depend on practice nurses' monitoring activities to inform their plans for a patient's care.

There is a third dimension to this approach to nursing 'care' which is particularly relevant in the light of recent policy emphases on the service user's 'voice' and care as 'partnership' with 'patients' (DH, 1989a, 1994). Particularly because this task-orientated and 'conveyor belt' approach (Pursey, 1992) to practice is undertaken within an organizational context which is financially driven, the interactions with clients are also strictly bounded in time. Fixed and highly limited amounts of clinic and/or nurses' time are allocated to the completion of each task. For immunizations and blood pressure checks, it may be as little as 5 minutes. For cervical smears it may be 15 minutes. Nurses feel that there is no time to embark upon a detailed conversation, and therefore limit opportunities for clients to divulge information and details about themselves which do not pertain to the specific, and arguably narrowly conceived, issue in hand. The strictly bounded purpose and the time limits of the client–nurse interaction therefore militate against the client having much, if any, 'leverage' on the interaction itself. Indeed, clients' clues, tentatively proffered, about their own concerns were often observed to be ignored or 'unheard' by the nurse during these busy interactions. The focus for the interaction is therefore the body and a physical or medical condition rather than the person and his or her circumstances. For example, practice nurses vaccinating young children in clinics rarely attempted to address parenting or child development issues during the interaction. This may be because of the nurse's own recognition that she does not possess the requisite training or skills or because of the tight time-tabling of the self-financing clinics, which ensures maximum throughput for minimum cost. Clients interviewed during the study were very understanding of the pressures of time under which nurses were working in this context (Westlake and Pearson, 1995a, 1995b), and other studies have shown that where alternative services are available which enable the specific task to be completed within an organizational framework which allows more time for 'listening', some clients prefer to use such a service (Pearson *et al.*, 1991).

Nursing as an holistic, integrated process

In the holistic approach to nursing practice, the nurse takes account of the client as a person in his or her broader socio-economic context, integrating a wider range of component parts of 'care' in her practice. The focus is on the development of the nurse–client relationship, the continuity and intensity of which is valued and concentrated upon by the nurse. This approach to nursing care was most commonly observed among district nurses (DNs) and health visitors for older people (HVOP), most of whom saw their clients principally in their own homes about long-term problems and conditions. In this framework, PHC nurses consider their practice to be effective only where their relationship with the client is underpinned by trust and support. The social interaction and quality of the relationship between the client and nurse is therefore as important as any functional activity. Some nurses visit clients in order to 'keep an eye' on them, or to maintain contact with them, often 'doing' something whilst they are there, such as helping a client fill out a form or to organize their medicines, which helps to maintain the relationship.

This holistic approach to nursing 'care' involves a continuous, long-term process, in strong contrast to discrete, episodic contacts with an immediate agenda and strictly bounded purpose. Through such continuous involvement, which varies in intensity, the nurse builds up an understanding of a client's situation, which rarely remains static. She is thereby able to assess changes in the client's circumstances, to which she can respond with anticipatory and preventive strategies. This is particularly applicable to older people living at home who, despite becoming more frail, are eager to maintain their independence (Westlake and Pearson, 1995b) and to families with young children who are under increasing stress with problems of unemployment and poor housing and need support with child care and parenting (Westlake and Pearson, 1995a). It was also observed to be a key aspect of district nursing sisters' care of people who were terminally ill: they frequently described their regular visits to assess the situation as 'keeping an eye on them', anticipating that greater nursing involvement would be required at a later stage. The PHC nurses who adopt this approach to their work tend to be concerned with individual clients' general circumstances and overall health status as well as any immediate and specific health problems. The problems addressed therefore have more of a psychological and social component than those addressed by the task-orientated approach and clients are encouraged to share their concerns, worries and feelings with the nurse. One older woman, who became very tearful and upset, indicated that her family probably had no idea that she felt as depressed and alone as she had revealed to the HVOP. This approach draws on the nurse's specialist psychological, social and socio-environmental knowledge, which often results in them receiving referrals direct from other primary care professionals who may not have the requisite knowledge and breadth of understanding about the issues involved or access to the necessary resources and networks.

This holistic approach to PHC nursing care thus emphasizes the nurse's role as a 'supporter' rather than a 'doer', so that the nature and boundaries of nursing care are less clearly defined. In these cases, the nurses are more likely to work with other professionals as autonomous equals in collaboration, rather than as a 'subsidiary' member of a GP's support team. In some cases, as a result of her knowledge and contacts, the PHC nurse may refer her clients directly on to another professional or service such as social services or to a specialist health service, such as a mental illness service, rather than suggest that they return to the GP who may then refer them.

During these interactions, tensions could arise between a nurse's own conceptualization of appropriate care and statutory policy imperatives. The prime example is in respect of health visitors with child protection responsibilities who recognized the crucial importance in their health visiting practice of establishing trust with parents and families, and support them in their parenting, but, where the safety of a child was in question, are required by the paramountcy of the child's interests (Fox Harding, 1991a, 1991b) to take the ultimate and unilateral decision about the situation, thereby risking the betrayal of the parents' trust (Westlake and Pearson, 1995a). Similarly, health visitors working with older people whose health and personal circumstances were deteriorating, or had reached crisis point, were observed to negotiate skilfully the tensions between the client's wishes to remain independent at home and the health visitor's concerns for the older person's welfare and safety.

This holistic approach to PHC nursing had several key features. First, it usually involved considerable dialogue between the client and nurses. In contrast to the mechanistic, biomedical, task-orientated approach, clients were encouraged to disclose and discuss their worries and fears, some of which could be significant issues, and the nurse encouraged the involvement of others in the household. This discussion and exchange of information during the interaction increased the nurse's understanding of the client's situation, constraints and opportunities to effect change. The nurse's care was therefore observed to have more relevance to the client's own circumstances and perceived needs. Second, the nature of the nurse's practice and relationship with a specific client evolved over time, during repeated and continuous contact often after having, in the first instance, made contact to perform a specific and narrowly defined clinical task or assessment. Third, interactions between nurses and clients were more likely to be in the clients' home than in a clinic or health centre. Fourth, the process and outcome of these interactions were usually intangible and difficult to define and measure, and were inadequately summarized in the categories available in current management information systems (Flynn et al., 1995; Hiscock and Pearson, 1996). Nurses taking this approach were often concerned with the process of care giving, and with clients' perceptions of their work rather than with any immediate or long-term outcome.

'Care' in the primary health care nursing market

Our research demonstrates there is no single concept of care in PHC nursing. Nursing care in primary health care settings is as diverse as the subdivisions and subspecialties themselves, yet PHC nurses are increasingly treated by policy documents and managers as a single professional group, representing a unified nursing resource which can be deployed to maximum cost-effectiveness by substituting for each other as required (NHSME, 1993). The diversity of concepts and practice of care in PHC nursing resonate with the debate (Thomas, 1993) about the components of 'care' as being split into caring activities and feeling or emotional aspects, a distinction which, although somewhat artificial, has been characterized as 'caring for' and 'caring about' or as 'physical' and 'emotional' labour (James, 1992).

It is evident from our data that practice nurse care is dominated by the performance of delegated functional tasks or caring activities which are often highly technical, with clearly drawn boundaries, resulting in limited scope for clients to influence the agenda. Our data also indicate that the organizational and policy context of practice nurses' work affords little scope for 'caring about' clients in the sense of emotional labour and involvement.

There is considerable dispute about which tasks GPs should be permitted to transfer to practice nurses, who have been criticized for undertaking what some nurses claim to be 'doctors' work'. One author suggested that the appropriateness of delegated tasks should be determined by whether the task improves nursing practice or creates a competent physician's assistant (Hobbs and Stilwell, 1990). The question of what should or should not be delegated to practice nurses reflects disagreements about the professional status of nursing and what constitutes the 'essence' of nursing care, but the policy agenda within the UK dictates that the relationship between GPs and practice nurses operates on the basis of employer–employee. This gives situational power to the GP who can determine the boundaries of practice nurses' work. GPs have a responsibility to ensure that contractual requirements set out at policy level are satisfied, and to a large extent they rely on practice nurses to undertake delegated tasks on their behalf. Health policy and contractual responsibilities for delivery of services are thus interpreted through the frame of reference of the medical profession, which is essentially orientated to the detection and treatment of illness and disease rather than to the broader and more positive concept of health (WHO, 1981, 1985). Whilst some authors criticize nurses who practice within a 'medical' framework for reducing the patient to the status of a condition (McIntosh, 1977; Menzies, 1970), the other argument is that nurses focus on psychosocial aspects of care at the expense of physical care and thereby deny one of their key functions.

Practice nurses are undoubtedly a highly heterogeneous group and their work is highly context-specific (Pursey, 1992). Given that they are expected to undertake a wide range of functions and tasks delegated by their GP employees (Greenfield *et al.*, 1987) their levels of autonomy and responsibility can be expected to vary according to their level of expertise, competence and professional interests. The diversity of practice nursing work (Hirst *et al.*, 1995) and the somewhat *ad hoc* development of the nurse practitioner role in the UK demonstrate how fluid and flexible practice nurses are able to be. Unlike health visitors or district nurses who have their own professionally determined definition of legitimate areas of practice, they are more able to respond rapidly to the external context of changing policy agendas, organizational arrangements and management requirements. This flexibility and the ability of their nursing 'care' to be measured quantitatively strengthens their market position within the rapidly changing mixed economy of the reformed NHS.

By comparison, health visitors consider their 'caring' to be about meeting the psychological, social and environmental needs of families and children and, where relevant, older people. For health visitors, 'health' is defined predominantly within a social environmental model, with a clear acknowledgement that a person's physical health is embodied in his or her emotional and social well-being and the environment within which he or she lives (WHO, 1981; 1985). Health is seen not as a physical 'steady state' but as a constant, ongoing process. For health visitors, 'care' is therefore conceptualized as the emotional labour of 'caring about' people's lives over time and has a dimension of continuity embedded within it, although they also care 'for' clients in some organizational contexts by undertaking some functional tasks in clinics such as developmental checks and giving immunizations. The individual is therefore seen as having a vital role in shaping and taking control over life-choices and decisions about health. Health visitors perceive caring as involving an 'empowerment' process and giving people the skills and knowledge with which to effect change and take responsibility for their own health. Health visitors for older people, in particular, focused on primary prevention of potential health problems by trying to reduce the impact of risk factors in older people, such as poor safety in households. It is within this model of care and the work associated with it that the clearest overlap with 'social care' can be observed (Pearson and Wistow, 1995).

Of all the professional subdisciplines within what we have termed primary health care nursing, health visiting has perhaps been the most threatened by the NHS reforms. Exploratory research suggests that GP fundholders in particular are questioning the value and purpose of health visiting practice within the PHC team. Health visitors' work is being shifted away from person-orientated domiciliary visits to task-orientated sessions in child health clinics (Hiscock and Pearson, 1996). It has been suggested that it is easy to see why health visiting activity may not be highly valued by general managers, given its focus on 'nebulous' concepts such as family care (Fatchett, 1990). It does not 'fit' comfortably within the current policy and managerial emphasis on measurables, cost-effectiveness and value for money, as its outcomes are not easily defined, circumscribed or measured. In the late 1980s Orr (1988) expressed concern about the trend for other community-based nurses (mainly district nurses) to assert their superiority over health visitors. They were, she suggested, able to deliver what the GPs, general managers and consumers knew about and wanted, whereas confusion continued regarding the role and value of health visiting activity.

Our research suggests that it is district nurses who have most successfully managed to marry the external market demands for efficiency, value for money and outcome-related evidence of activity with the need to perceive patients within an holistic framework. Senior district nurses who are team leaders bemoan the fact that their role as managers leaves them little time for this approach, with the result that it is junior DNs and DN auxiliaries who adopt the most 'integrated' approach to care. This combination of attention to 'physical need', whilst establishing a relationship over time which facilitates the realization of the client–carer agenda, is where the district nurses' greatest strength seems to lie. They appear relatively unthreatened by GP fundholding, as they are able to develop strong alliances with GPs through the complementary (as opposed to delegated) tasks they undertake with clients, which reflects a traditional hospital model of nursing in which the district nurse could be likened to the ward sister. District nurses appear to operationalize their concept of care through something similar to Maslow's (1970) hierarchy of need, where the basic physical needs of patients (caring 'for') are met alongside the expressive, affective behaviours demonstrated through the nurses' interactions (caring 'about'). For district nurses, physical care comes first, in that it is their first point of interaction with the client. The psychosocial interaction comes subsequently through the continued provision of that physical care and the establishment of an ongoing relationship with a client or family over time.

The market: thwarting diversity and choice?

Care is the concept through which nursing activity is often defined (Benner and Wrubel, 1989), although nurses use the term 'care' in many divergent and potentially contradictory ways (Kuhse, 1995). What is meant by 'nursing' and who is entitled to be called a 'nurse' changes over time and according to place and context (Wright and Hearn, 1993), prompting suggestions that we should refer to 'nursings'. There are also 'different ways of being a nurse' (Carpenter, 1980), so that no single or universal conceptualization of 'care' is likely within the profession. Our research demonstrates that there are shared features (Cash, 1990) in the ways that nurses conceptualize and operationalize their caring activities, although there are also some marked differences.

Clearly, there is no one *ideal* place for PHC nurses to be located on the continuum of care between the biomedical and the psychosocial. Rather, the diverse needs of people living within the community who have contact with PHC nurses for different purposes require different approaches and responses which, in turn, each have their place, function and value within the current spectrum of PHC nursing care. However, the structures and culture of the internal NHS market may well favour the task-orientated style of PHC nursing practice and thus nursing care, more than others. If this is the case, the apparently relentless and mechanistic 'logic' of the internal market will thwart one of its avowed aims: of affording people greater choice and ensuring services which better meet their needs.

Endnotes

4.1 Throughout this chapter, we use the term 'primary health care' to refer to the range of settings, outside hospitals and nursing homes, in which health care is delivered, including community-based clinics, people's own homes and general medical practitioners' surgeries.

4.2 In this chapter, we use the term 'PHC nurse(s)' to refer to the range of nurses working in primary health care settings who were included in our empirical study: practice nurses; health visitors; health/nurse visitors for older people; and district nurses who included 'qualified', registered nurses and auxiliary nurses who may have had some training but did not possess formal professional qualifications.

4.3 General and specialist (for example, psychiatric nursing, continence advice, stoma care) nursing services provided in 'community' settings outside hospitals by nurses employed by community health service providers and not employed directly by GPs.

4.4 In the UK, general medical care is organized within the publicly-funded NHS by individuals being 'registered' with a specific doctor or group of doctors by whom all their primary medical care is delivered. Only in exceptional circumstances (such as being on holiday or a temporary resident) can such people receive medical care from an NHS GP with whom they are not registered.

4.5 We would expect the issues discussed to apply also to more specialist nurses working in primary health care whose position may be even more threatened by the increasing fragmentation of service commissioning and purchasing and the associated reluctance to contract jointly for specialist services across health districts.

4.6 Throughout the chapter we use the term 'client' rather than 'patient' because the latter implies that people are ill and have adopted a sick role. Many of the people with whom PHC nurses are concerned are not specifically ill as such, although within practice nursing the term 'patient' is most frequently used.

4.7 All the nurses included in this study were women.

References

Badger, F., Cameron, E. and Evers, H. 1989: The nursing auxiliary service and the care of elderly patients. *Journal of Advanced Nursing* **14**, 471–7.

Benner, P. and Wrubel, J. 1989: *The primacy of caring: stress and coping in health and illness.* Menlo Park, CA: Addison-Wesley.

Bennett, C. and Ferlie, E. 1994: Management by contract: rhetoric or reality? Some evidence from the NHS. Paper presented to the ERU conference, Cardiff, September.

BGS/HVA 1986: *Health visiting for the health of the aged. a joint policy statement.* London: British Geriatric Society/Health Visitors Association.

Carpenter, M. 1980: Asylum nursing before 1914: a chapter in the history of labour. In Davies, C. (ed.), *Rewriting nursing history.* London: Croom Helm 123–46.

Cash, K. 1990: Nursing models and the idea of nursing. *International Journal of Nursing* **27**(3), 249–56.

de la Cuesta, C. 1992: *Marketing the service: basic social process in health visiting.* Unpublished PhD thesis. Liverpool: University of Liverpool.

DH 1986: *Neighbourhood nursing.* The Cumberledge Report. Department of Health. London: HMSO.

DH 1989a: *Working for patients.* Department of Health. London: HMSO.

DH 1989b: *General practice in the NHS: a new contract.* Department of Health. London: HMSO.

DH 1989c: *Caring for people*. Cm 849, Department of Health. London: HMSO.

DH 1992: *Health of the nation: a strategy for health in England*. Cm 1986, Department of Health. London: HMSO.

DH 1993: *Research for health*. Department of Health. London: HMSO.

DH 1994: Developing NHS purchasing and GP fundholding, EL(94)79. London: Department of Health.

DH 1995a: *Health and personal social services statistics for England*, 1995 Edn, Department of Health. London: HMSO.

DHSS 1981: *Growing older*. Department of Health and Social Security. London: HMSO.

DHSS 1987: *Promoting better health: the government's programme for improving primary health care*. Cm 249, Department of Health and Social Security. London: HMSO.

Fatchett, A.B. 1990: Health visiting: a withering profession? *Journal of Advanced Nursing* **15**, 216–22.

Ferlie, E. 1994: The creation and evolution of quasi-markets in the public sector: early evidence from the NHS. *Policy and Politics* **22**(2), 105–12.

Flynn, R., Pickard, S. and Williams, G. 1995: Contracts and the quasi-market in community health services. *Journal of Social Policy* **24**(4), 529–50.

Freemantle, N., Watt, I. and Mason, J. 1993: Developments in the purchasing process in the NHS: towards an explicit politics of rationing? *Public Administration* **71**, 535–48.

Fox Harding, L. 1991a: The Children Act 1989 in context: four perspectives in child care law and policy (I). *Journal of Social Welfare and Family Law* **2**, 179–93.

Fox Harding, L. 1991b: The Children Act 1989 in context: four perspectives in child care law and policy (II). *Journal of Social Welfare and Family Law* **2**, 194–201.

Greenfield, S., Stilwell, B. and Drury, M. 1987: Practice nurses: social and occupational characteristics. *Journal of Royal College of General Practitioners* **37**, 341–5.

Ham, C. 1992: *Health policy in Britain*. London: Macmillan.

Harris, A. 1992: Health checks for people over 75. *British Medical Journal* **305**, 599–600.

Hirst, M., Atkin, K. and Lunt, N. 1995: Variations in practice nursing. *Health and Social Care in the Community* **3**(2), 83–97.

Hiscock, J. and Pearson, M. 1996: Professional costs and invisible value: the market in community nursing. *Journal of Interprofessional Care* **10**(1), 23–31.

Hobbs, R. and Stilwell, B. 1990: The developing role of the practice nurse in Great Britain. In Stilwell, B. and Hobbs, R. (eds) *Nursing in general practice: clinical care*. Oxford: Radcliffe Medical Press.

James, N. 1992: Care = organisation + physical labour + emotional labour. *Sociology of Health and Illness* **14**(2), 488–509.

Kuhse, K. 1995: Clinical ethics and nursing: 'Yes' to caring, but 'No' to a female ethics of care. *Bioethics* **9**(3/4), 207–19.

Luker, K. and Orr, J. 1992: *Health visiting: towards community health nursing*. Oxford: Blackwell Scientific Publications.

McIntosh, I. 1977: *Communication and awareness in a cancer ward*. London: Croom Helm.

Maslow, A.H. 1970: *Motivation and personality*. New York: Harper and Row.

Menzies, N. 1970: *Communication and stress: a nursing perspective*. London: Macmillan.

NHSME 1992: Guidance on the extension of the hospital and community health services elements of the GP fundholding scheme from 1 April 1993. London: National Health Service Management Executive.

NHSME 1993: Nursing in primary health care: new world, new opportunities. London: National Health Service Management Executive.

Nocon, A. 1992: Old age benefit. *Health Service Journal* 16 July, 28–9.

Orr, J. 1988: Enemies of project 2000. *Nursing Times* **84**(44), 24.

Pearson, M., Spencer, S. and McKenna, M. 1991: Patterns of uptake and problems presented at well woman clinics in Liverpool. *Journal of Public Health Medicine* **13**(1), 42–7.

Pearson, M. and Wistow, G. 1995: The boundary between health and social care. *British Medical Journal* **311**, 208–9.

Pursey, A.C. 1992: *A comparison of health visitors' and practice nurses' constructions of work with older people in the community.* Unpublished PhD thesis. Liverpool: University of Liverpool.

Quinney, D. and Pearson, M. 1996: Different worlds, missed opportunities? Primary health care nursing in a north western health district. Liverpool: Health and Community Care Research Unit, University of Liverpool.

Reed, J. 1989: *All dressed up and nowhere to go: nursing assessment in geriatric care.* Unpublished PhD thesis. Newcastle-upon-Tyne: Newcastle-upon-Tyne Polytechnic.

Thomas, C. 1993: De-constructing concepts of care. *Sociology* **27**(4), 649–69.

Turner, B.S. 1992: *Regulating bodies: essays in medical sociology.* London: Routledge.

Waters, K. 1991: *The nurse's role in the rehabilitation of elderly people in hospital.* Unpublished PhD thesis. Manchester: University of Manchester.

Waterworth, S. and Luker, K. 1990: Reluctant collaborators: do patients want to be involved in decisions concerning care? *Journal of Advanced Nursing* **15**, 971–6.

Westlake, D. and Pearson, M. 1995a: Invisibly responsible? Managing health in households with young children. Liverpool: Health and Community Care Research Unit, University of Liverpool.

Westlake, D. and Pearson, M. 1995b: Maximising independence, minimising risk: older people's management of their health. Liverpool: Health and Community Care Research Unit, University of Liverpool.

Wilkinson, M.J. 1995: Love is not a marketable commodity: new public management in the British National Health Service. *Journal of Advanced Nursing* **21**, 980–7.

WHO 1981: *Health for all by the year 2000: a global strategy for health.* Geneva: World Health Organisation.

WHO 1985: *Targets for health for all.* Copenhagen, World Health Organisation Europe.

Wright, C.J. and Hearn, J. 1993: The 'invisible' man in nursing. Paper presented to the conference on Nursing, Women's History and the Politics of Welfare, University of Nottingham, Nottingham, July.

5

Health sector reform and profession power, autonomy and culture: the case of Australian allied health professions

Rosalie A. Boyce

Introduction

A preoccupation with health care reform has been a feature of industrialized countries in the 1990s. So constant is health reform activity that Saltman and von Otter (1995, p. 1) described it as 'part of the daily political landscape in much of Europe'. From a global perspective, the convergence of policy instruments to affect health care reform has generally centred around the mix of competition and regulation in the form of 'managed competition' and 'planned markets' (Ham *et al.*, 1990).

Greater regulation is being used by traditionally market-orientated systems, whilst those countries that have historically relied on centrally planned and regulated approaches (of which Australia is one) are implementing more competitive models of financing and delivery of health care services. Scott (1993), in an analysis of the main trajectories of change in the post-Second World-War US health care system, identified the commodification of health, the reduction in solo and small group provider organizations and the rise of managerial influence over professional influence as some of the key factors of change. Scott concluded that aside from the greater involvement of government regulatory activity, the nature of the changes reduced the uniqueness of health care from other sectors of economic activity.

At an institutional level the reform agenda is typically underpinned by moves to replace professional judgement on resource allocation with more rationally based managerial decision-making, such that the professionals responsible for resource expenditure are more accountable for their activities. It is in the institutional domain that the politicization of care and debates about clients as accounting principles affecting the hospitals' 'bottom line' are most transparent.

It is also in institutions such as hospitals that interprofessional conflict about the dominance of particular philosophies of care in an environment of scarce financial resources are most predictable (Robb, 1975). This is particularly the case as the organizational restructuring of hospitals based on models of devolving decision-making and financial management to clinical units brings the contest for resources closer to the clinical domain and the patient interface (Packwood *et al.*, 1991).

The purpose of this chapter is to demonstrate the increasing importance of factors related to the organizational domain in which health professional work is conducted to the power and autonomy of the professions and the construction of 'care'. The Australian allied health professions and their experience of health system reform and organizational restructuring is an excellent vehicle for studying the nature of change, opportunity and threat and the strategic response of numerically small specialist professions. But first one must deal with the question of who and what are the allied health professions and situate them in an international context.

Doctors, nurses and 'others': making the invisible visible

Research on the allied health professions in a cross-national context is hindered by a lack of definitional clarity. An examination of the literature shows that the term 'allied health' has been applied to an array of occupational groupings. These include Third World health workers through to higher degree professionals. In some settings, the nursing profession may also be referred to as an allied health profession. For the purposes of this chapter, interest lies with the professional segment of the disciplines and occupations variously assembled under the allied health rubric. Typically, this would correspond to occupations trained to at least the level of baccalaureate or university undergraduate degree.

From the Australian perspective, this would define the allied health professions as at least the rehabilitation or therapy professions (physiotherapy, occupational therapy, speech pathology), social work, psychology, dietetics, pharmacy, podiatry, audiology, medical librarians, prosthetics and orthotics, orthoptics, radiography and medical laboratory science. Data from a recent national census show that of the total workforce in health and health-related occupations, approximately 16 per cent is employed in allied health occupations using the Australian Council of Allied Health Professions membership criteria (ABS, 1991).

Although these disciplines represent a broad interpretation of the allied health professions, in some institutional settings only five or six professions may be considered as allied health professions in terms of management structures. In such a scenario, the core allied health professions almost always include physiotherapy, occupational therapy, speech pathology, social work, psychology, dietetics and pharmacy. Nursing in Australia is not considered as, nor does it consider itself to be, an allied health profession.

A history of direct management of radiography and medical laboratory science by the medical profession (radiology and pathology) results in these groups rarely participating in formal organizational allied health structures in Australian hospitals, although they are considered as allied health professions (Gardner and McCoppin, 1995). This is in contrast to the other named disciplines which have more typically been organized under an arrangement of profession hierarchies headed by a profession manager who formally reports to a medical director; a salaried executive-level medical appointment with no direct clinical service role (Duckett *et al.*, 1981; Boyce, 1991). A selected review of comparative discipline classifications in major Australian hospitals suggests that between 15 and 20 per cent of staff rendering direct patient care services are allied health professionals (Boyce, 1993a).

Describing or defining the allied health professions – what's in a name?

A major review of the US allied health workforce in the late 1980s by the Institute of Medicine, which attempted to define allied health comprehensively in terms of shared tasks and labour-market characteristics, was viewed as a generally unsatisfactory exercise (Institute of Medicine, 1989). The Institute of Medicine noted that although there was some dissatisfaction about the term 'allied health', the only consensus reached was a universal distaste for the predecessor term [paramedical]. It concluded (p. 17) that it was better not to attempt to generate a more precise definition of allied health:

> It is more important for pragmatism to continue to prevail and for old and new groups to draw what benefits they can from belonging to *allied health* than it is to have an accurate description of common characteristics that define the group.

The situation in Australia is similar and the term 'paramedical' is rarely used, particularly in formal documentation. The application of acceptable descriptors in relation to the health professions is a sensitive issue not only in terms of self-perceptions of influence but also in terms of cultural authority. Safriet (1994, p. 313) has demonstrated the nature of the sensitivity and its implications for influence in a condemnation of policy-makers' use of terms such as 'non-physician providers' and 'physician extender': 'By making physicians the norm and identifying these other providers only as not-physicians, or less-than-physicians, we render culturally invisible the fine contribution they have been making all along'.

The bulk of prior research on the allied health professions has concentrated on studies of the individual professions and represents a focus on internal analysis and developing a sense of the 'uniqueness' of the specialty. The focus on the internal, and in particular a preoccupation with whether the discipline is a profession, how it can be more professional or reach the status of a 'true' profession continue to appear with regularity in profession-sponsored journals (Bruhn, 1993; Collins, 1993; Sachs and Labovitz 1994; Schemm, 1993). This is despite extensive agreement in the sociological literature over the past two decades that trait-based approaches are of very limited utility. Although more critical approaches have appeared in some profession-sponsored journals (Hugman, 1991a; Irvine and Graham, 1994) they continue to be rare. The nursing profession, more than the allied health professions, has embraced a more critical approach, in part because of a greater acceptance of the insights brought through feminist theory and critical approaches which question professionalism as an instrument of patriarchal domination (Davies, 1995a; Porter, 1992; Wicks, 1995; Witz, 1994).

The concentration on studying individual allied health professions has obscured the notion of 'allied health' as a cultural phenomenon and a strategic resource. My own study of different approaches to organizing the allied health professions in Australian general hospitals showed that an 'allied health' subculture can emerge from the shared experience of medical authority, organizational isolation and the social experience of being a non-medical and non-nursing profession in a complex organization (Boyce, 1996).

The use of the term 'allied health' to describe, but not necessarily to define, a diverse set of health providers has become increasing institutionalized in Australia. The argument is not that the allied health professions are homogeneous from an applied technology or task perspective. Rather, the contention is that in terms of social relations, particularly in terms of the relationships with medicine and more broadly within key organizational settings, the allied health professions occupy a similar location in terms of the division of labour and their isolation from sources of power (Boyce, 1996). From this perspective, the overarching concept of medical dominance continues to be an important theoretical and structural element in a contemporary understanding of the position of the allied health professions.

Health reform: the implications for allied health professionals

The medical profession has been the target of most reformist activity and the profession on which most research has been undertaken. A key focus of analysis has been the extent to which the raft of policy and procedural approaches introduced to manage clinical activity more explicitly will produce a diminution, if any, of medical power (Begun and Lippincott, 1993; Flynn, 1992; Hafferty and McKinlay, 1993; Harrison and Pollitt, 1994).

Whilst commentators trade examples arguing for and against a shift in the substantive position of medicine, the other health professions, with the exception of nursing (Keen and Malby, 1992; Robinson *et al.*, 1992), remain almost invisible in the terms of analysis. Although little is known about the distinct issues which the allied health professions face within the context of reformist activity there is no reason to assume that they will be immune to the impact of relentless pressures for reform (Blayney and Fitz, 1990; Boyce, 1991, 1993a; Larkin, 1988; Øvretveit, 1992, 1994; Berry, 1994).

The specific demographics of the allied health professions has acted to protect them to some extent from being identified as a primary target for reformist zeal. As individual disciplines, their small numerical size makes them less likely candidates for intensive scrutiny because they do not represent a significant level of expenditure within total national outlays on health. The focus on medicine and nursing as the primary targets of reform has enveloped the allied health professions with a degree of anonymity which has avoided the direct attention of economizers. However, the low levels of political activity and organizational infrastructure of the allied health professions, together with their history of relying on the protection of medicine and their lack of attention to strategic-level issues, makes them vulnerable to adverse outcomes (Begun and Lippincott, 1993; Boyce, 1991).

Larkin (1988) contended that it would be difficult to conclude that the forces affecting the autonomy of the medical profession would not have even further-reaching effects on the less-powerful health professions. A crucial issue, at least from the perspective of the allied health professions, is whether the thrust of the reformist project fortifies or displaces the premier position of medicine in authority relations within the division of labour. An alternative prediction, and one which has been observed in some British analyses such as those by Øvretveit (1994), Lloyd-Smith (1995) and Young (1995), is that more competitive approaches to health care and the penetration of internal market reforms may provide new opportunities for the allied health professions through the operation of 'business autonomy' as a new form of organizationally-mediated professional independence. Similar predictions have been made in relation to the organizational reform of the Australian health care system, although there has not been the length of experience with competitive reforms as has been evident in the experience of the United Kingdom and other European countries (Boyce 1993a, 1995; Harrison, 1995; Saltman and von Otter, 1995).

The impact of systemwide and institutional-level change on the health professions and how they negotiate the 'business' of care against a background of greater competition and managerialism has been the subject of analysis. What is most striking about the research to date is its primarily medico-centric nature (Flynn, 1992; Giaimo, 1995; Harrison, 1995) with a lesser consideration on the nursing profession (Ackroyd, 1995; Davies, 1995b; Keen and Malby, 1992; Witz, 1994) and the seemingly invisible status of the many other health professions which constitute our understanding of the 'multidisciplinary' nature of modern health care.

Hugman (1991b, p. 60) drew a link between the 'semi-marginalized' status of the British remedial therapies and their neglect of the importance of organizational issues:

> It appears probable that the structural location of the remedial therapies is reflected in the inattention to organisational and structural issues in the writings of remedial therapists, and the relative ignoring of remedial therapists in academic studies of organisation, in comparison either to nursing or to social work.

The lack of a highly placed executive manager at the institutional level for the remedial professions was also identified by Hugman (1991b) as a factor in the relative powerlessness of the professions. Similarly, the Institute of Medicine (1989, p. 219), in a major Congress-mandated study of allied health personnel in the United States, contended that the lack of an 'umbrella allied health administrator position to promote the interests and raise the level of visibility of the allied health work force' reduced their influence.

Contests of control – clinicians, clinical work and core business functions

Part of the struggle over the recognition of a more pluralist construction of interest in the impact of health care reform, at least as it has been transacted in Australia, has occurred in relation to the understanding of the term 'clinician'. The preservation of 'clinician' as a taken-for-granted synonym for doctor is under challenge and, in the context of the Australian situation, is generally conceded to be a multidisciplinary term.[5.1] There are similar arguments over the notion of 'clinical work' as an synonym for doctor's work.

The non-medical professions' interest in the definitional parameters for policy and operational purposes of 'clinician' is clear. The opportunity for the inclusion of profession-based interest groups in shaping the operational and implementational context of reform depends to some extent on the recognition of the group as a legitimate stakeholder and influential political entity. If the non-medical professions are to achieve influence, if not in the framing and propagation of new policy then at least in its operational context, then they must make the case for their fundamental role in defining and managing clinical care as part of specifying their connection to core business functions. Further, they must be able to make a nexus between this role and their ability to act as effective and strategic resource and cost managers. These points of control represent important profession resources which Hickson *et al.* (1971) argued, in their strategic contingency theory of intraorganizational power, are related to subunit (or profession) power through their ability to cope with uncertainty, substitutability and organizational centrality. Hence it is not surprising that the contest in the clinical domain about the nature of a clinician and clinical work are often most clearly evident in the struggle over governance structures during organizational restructuring (ANF, 1991; Boyce, 1991).

It has been predicted that it may only be the threat of negative outcomes arising from the restructuring of hospitals which galvanizes the allied health professions into more collaborative political approaches to resist organizational forms which the individual disciplines believe are antithetical to the aspirations of the professions in terms of their independence (Boyce, 1991; Gardner and McCoppin, 1995) .

Operating in the reformist agenda: the challenge of organization

Policy shifts associated with increasing managerialism and competition, and their impact on shaping policy and practice at the institutional level, have transformed the environment in which the allied health professions operate. New strategic arenas have arisen in which opportunities to expand their independence relative to the medical profession coexist with conditions which could lead to the non-medical professions being subject to greater medical (and managerial) control over their work. The ultimate shape of post-reform relations with the medical profession and the uptake of allied health's perspective on care and service priorities into policy frameworks and institutional procedures are intricately tied to their ability to gain influence in reform politics.

It is argued that there are two fundamental barriers to the allied health professions achieving greater influence in policy debates and maximizing their opportunities for participation in the direction and implementation of health sector reforms. First, there is the myopic concentration of the professions, and professionals, on the clinical domain of care at the expense of a wider appreciation of policy and organizational politics. Ignoring, or underestimating, the nature of transformational change at a systems level, particularly when it is fuelled by a convergence of policy and practice from a global perspective, is a perilous strategy to adopt, if indeed it could be described as a strategy. The nature of the hazard is no less when analysed from the perspective of the institutional level, where organizational restructuring affecting the traditional bases of power of the professions has become routine: 'Lack of knowledge about the consequences of organisational change resulting from restructuring and exclusion from a strategic influence in the process of change makes allied health professions vulnerable to a substantial reversal of both power and prospects' (Boyce, 1991, p. 150).

The second barrier has parallels with the first in that the 'tyranny of tribalism' in the allied health professions is an obstacle to achieving effective influence. Tribalism arrests the development of collective cross-profession positions on policy, particularly as it pertains to organizational or managerial issues. The continuation of individual profession-specific approaches produces a form of naive self-exclusion from policy processes. The allied health disciplines are faced with a pressing need to achieve a new level of aggregation, integration and, in some circumstances, social closure under the umbrella of 'allied health'.

The inherent difficulty, or unwillingness, of the allied health professions to respond to the cues and signals of policy-makers for more externally-focused and cross-profession approaches has been noted both by US and by British analysts. For example, Blayney and Fitz (1990, p. 8) argued in the context of the US health and education system that the large numbers of allied health occupational groupings and their primary identification with 'their' profession rather than the broader allied health grouping has produced a crisis of leadership and a concentration on 'tribes rather than on nations'. Similarly, from the British perspective both Beattie (1995) and Hugman (1995) have identified tribal boundaries of health and social service professions as a barrier to change.

The notion of 'tribes' and 'nations' is a useful metaphor for understanding the nature of responses to attempts by individual professions to penetrate policy processes. Policy-makers prefer to 'deal with' nations rather than multiple tribes where there is an inherent rationality to a collective approach within a cooperative environment. Where the nation is deemed to be uncooperative, a strategy to foster the development of a cooperative tribe to gain leverage over the nation is not uncommon.

In later sections of this chapter, the emergence of a number of national and state-based allied health organizations and events as a strategic response to the desire to participate in the Australian reform agenda (proactive and defensive responses) will be explored. These events represent a form of collective behaviour through strategic coalitions and networks of cooperation that were not evident in Australia prior to the 1990s.

In addition to these developments, a major site of contest over influence and professional power has occurred over the implementation of new organizational forms as part of hospital restructuring. New organizational models have implications for the expansion and contraction of the power and autonomy of the allied health professions, particularly as some models eliminate profession-based departments whereas other models are consistent with greater self-management at the corporate level (Boyce, 1992).

It is argued that the opportunity for allied-health-determined concepts of 'care' to be implemented without the distortion of medical constructions of what is appropriate for allied health vary in part according to the structural conditions inherent in different organizational models. And further, these changes in institutional-level arrangements which place the allied health professions in new configurations of interdependence act on the development of an 'allied health profession community' subculture.

In the following section I trace the development of 'allied health' as a recognized entity at national, state and regional levels. The beginnings of the allied health professions' collective participation in a broad range of policy and procedural developments are evident from these developments. In addition, the emergence of allied health as a recognizable entity provides the collective consultation framework which government and policy-makers have been seeking (Macklin, 1992; NHSU, 1991a).

I will follow this with an in-depth examination of the pivotal implications for the allied health professions from the reform agenda in the organizational design of public hospitals and the emergence of new forms of allied health organization at the workplace level.

'Allied health' as a recognizable entity

A feature of the 1990s has been the emergence of the Australian allied health professions as a distinct organizational entity. In the language of policy-makers, 'allied health' has assumed the status of a comfortable and efficient umbrella term for including the multiple health professions outside medicine and nursing. This has particularly been the case since the beginning of the major Australian health strategy review period associated with the work of the National Health Strategy Unit from 1990–93 (du Toit, 1995; Gardner and McCoppin, 1995). Less certain has been the comfort level of the disciplines understood to constituent 'allied health' in adapting to an institutional and policy environment which increasingly expects them to operate as a collective unit.

As the impact of system-wide and institutional-level change has started to bite, the allied health professions have attempted to find mechanisms through which to participate. A crucial part of their attempts to penetrate the crowded market place of political influence has been to reconfigure the nature of relationships *between* the disciplines that constitute the 'allied health' rubric into a more collaborative approach. This strategy has been most evident in the organizational domain of the public-sector acute-care general hospital through the operation of divisions of allied health (Boyce, 1992).

Outside the institutional level, the emergence of 'allied health' as a policy-relevant entity has been less uniform and this is partly explained by the lack of an infrastructure capable of supporting the national communications framework necessary to achieve effective participation in a country approximately 30 times the size of the United Kingdom and with a population double that of London. Consequently, much of the energy and drive behind the emergence of 'allied health' has occurred at the institutional and regional level, a factor which will be explored in greater depth in later sections of the chapter.

The development of local 'allied health' power bases and champions nested within the relative security of leadership positions within large general hospitals in the public sector has had an impact on the development of allied health quasi-organizations and associations at a statewide and national level. In particular the emergence of a new organizational position such as the 'allied health director' has been a crucial factor in the development of a national leadership infrastructure that had previously been limited to a within-profession phenomenon.[52]

Institutional health care executives and government policy-makers have assisted in the emergence of favourable conditions supportive of the 'allied health' collective and allied health directors. This has occurred through their adoption of an inclusive stakeholder terminology of 'doctors, nurses and allied health' which has increasingly stressed their expectation of a collective position from the allied health professions. The influence of constructing 'allied health' as a collective entity and its impact on eliciting collective behaviour from the professions, particularly on organizational rather than clinical matters, should not be underestimated. For example, Furnham *et al.* (1981, p. 297) have demonstrated that decisions about the nature of separating and grouping health professions was sufficient to precipitate the 'psychological processes that lead to inter-group prejudice'.

National initiatives in allied health organization

The Australian Council of Allied Health Professionals (ACAHP) has been in existence for some 20 years. The Council is constituted by a representative from each of 14 different occupational classifications which have been accepted as allied health professions under their charter for membership. Its focus of activity has been largely restricted to providing input into the Australian Council of Health Care Standards (formerly the Australian Council of Hospital Standards, an organization devoted to voluntary accreditation of hospitals).

Despite more recent attempts to expand its ambit of influence, the ACAHP remains largely marginalized from policy debate or influence on operational issues at the institutional level. This lack of influence can be attributed in large part to its unwieldy structure of professional representation and the requirement for it to consult with the professions prior to developing or commenting on policy. Gardner and McCoppin (1995, p. 390) have concluded that despite the ACAHP being the obvious forum for influence, it has 'never realised its potential as a powerful, peak organisation in allied health'.

A turning point in the development of 'allied health' as a recognizable entity occurred in April 1992 with the conduct of the first National Allied Health Services Conference, 'Unity Through Diversity', which attracted in excess of 300 registrants from 19 different occupational classifications throughout all the states and territories of Australia. The importance of the allied health professions providing an accessible mechanism for communicating with key opinion leaders and government regulators was stressed at the conference by the director of the influential National Health Strategy Unit (Macklin, 1992). An outcome of the conference was the identification of a network of allied health directors and coordinators who elected to maintain contact on a regular basis and to form a working party to establish a national group or association (National Allied Health Management Group (NAHMG)) capable of representing the interests of allied health managers.

The attitude of the individual allied health profession associations towards the development of 'allied health' as an entity is both complex and paradoxical. On the one hand, the profession associations have supported the emergence of divisions of allied health under the leadership of a director of allied health within institutional settings such as hospitals or geographic regions. This is not surprising given that in the allied health division model the departmental structure of the profession is maintained under direct profession management, and an allied health director substituted (at a cheaper salary) for a medical director.

Less certain is the attitude of the profession associations to the emergence of an 'allied health' movement or organization at the national level in particular. Such organizations represent potential rivals to the profession associations because they are a logically attractive option for government and other policy-makers seeking single-point input into, or response to, policy development.

A survey of profession associations and relevant individuals towards the proposed formation of the NAHMG provides some an indication of attitudes. (Note that the membership of the NAHMG was to be based on individuals such as directors of allied health, not a council of professions models.) Analysis of the 134 respondents (81 individuals, 27 allied health profession associations and 18 health agencies or hospitals) to a discussion paper (NAHMGWP, 1993) showed that the national profession associations were the most likely to oppose the proposal. Another pattern in the data was the lack of consistency between the state and national offices of the same profession associations, with the states more likely to endorse the proposal. This result could be interpreted as a criticism of the national offices' performance in the areas which the NAHMG intended to pursue, for example, liaison with government agencies on 'allied health' matters.

Whilst some allied health profession associations appear to be opposed to the notion of an allied health association, the wish of government health departments to obtain 'allied health' input into policy and planning is a potential countervailing pressure capable of supporting further allied health developments (Macklin, 1992; NHSU, 1991). The patronage of the state through substantial funding of the special-purpose allied health groups discussed below is further evidence of the support for 'allied health' as an organizing principle.

Australian unions with coverage of the allied health professions have adopted a different position from profession associations on the emergence of 'allied health' as a recognizable entity. They have also been the most vigorous in their endorsement of allied health organizational structures in hospitals (Bremner, 1993; PSA, 1990). The role of industrial advocacy and representation of allied health workers in Australia is the preserve of unions rather than the allied health profession associations, and coverage is typically multidisciplinary. As a result, the relevant trade unions are less likely to be concerned about the emergence of multidisciplinary allied health associations. The unions are likely to support the emergence of a broad-based 'allied health' movement because, like government agencies, they share the desire to reduce the costly consultation overhead that negotiating with multiple small profession associations represents.

National developments in support of 'allied health' rather than discipline-specific activity has also occurred with funding support from the federal government through the Commonwealth Department of Human Services and Health. Since the early 1990s grants in excess of Aus$ 300 000 have been awarded to support the activity of newly formed quasi-associations such as the National Allied Health Casemix Committee and the National Allied Health Best Practice Consortium.[53] The Australian Allied Health Rural Health Taskforce has also received ongoing support for its activities and representative role on the Australian Rural Health Alliance.

In each case the public face of these organizations is unequivocally 'allied health' with discipline-based activities accommodated within the internal operating structure. Although no empirical studies have been conducted to measure trends in the success of allied health applications for competitive federal funding support, there is persuasive anecdotal evidence of increasing support for collaborative proposals from the allied health sector in a number of federal programme areas such as rural health, ambulatory care and casemix education and development.

State and regional initiatives in allied health organization

In addition to 'allied health' activity at the national level, there has also been significant development at the state level. Several allied health associations of various levels of formality have emerged to interact with government and promote allied health issues. Relevant examples include the Queensland Council of Allied Health Professions and the Tasmanian Health Professionals Council. Each of these bodies has a network of regional groups mirroring the boundaries of the relevant regional health authorities in their state, although in the case of the Queensland example the regional bodies are fully autonomous and in no formal relationship with the state-based body. The formation of these Councils occurred in the early 1990s and coincided with a period of very active reform of state health systems. Somewhat curiously, there are no formal or obvious informal links between the various state-based councils or with the ACAHP. And further, although the membership of the Councils are based on profession representation, there is wide variation in the occupational classifications of the constituent profession members.

These new forms of 'allied health' organization must be regarded as in a formative and emerging stage of development. Their persistence over several years, at varying levels of activity, despite the specific geographic constraints imposed by the size of Australia, indicate a certain resilience. It also suggests that they are meeting the needs of experienced allied health professionals in a manner which the individual profession associations have not been able to achieve. The diversity of organizations appearing may reflect the complexity of federal–state–local government relations in the provision of health care services. Effective political operation necessitates that the allied health professions organize to mirror the sites of government decision-making if their attempts at influence are to be effective.

Reforming the key site of health care production processes – the public hospital

In earlier parts of the chapter I have touched on the importance of institutional- or workplace-level organization of the allied health professions as an important factor in the expression of profession power and autonomy. In this context, the role of the hospital, and particularly the public hospital in Australia, is especially important as it is the public hospital which has experienced the most concerted attempts at reform through changes to organizational design and workplace relations (NHSU, 1993). A review of the rise of 'allied health' as an entity at national and state levels suggests that much of the energy and drive underpinning its development has been related to innovation and organizational change at the level of key worksites, in particular, public hospitals (Weeks, 1991).

The most common change in Australian public hospitals has been the implementation of devolved management and financial systems around clinical units by means of governance structures which incorporate leadership and management roles for medical clinician managers. A phenomenon observed in the early stages of restructuring was the myopic preoccupation of Australian health care executives on the UK Guy's Hospital model and the US Johns Hopkins Hospital model (Boyce, 1993b). The outcome of the rhetoric on restructuring for the allied health professions was a prevalent view among health care executives that profession-managed departments should be abandoned and the health professionals divided and directly employed by the clinical units (Boyce, 1991; Catchlove, 1991; Scarf, 1991). The prospect of an end to unified profession-managed services was regarded as a threat by allied health profession associations and unions (APA, 1994). If 'unity through diversity' was not an adequate stimulus to more collaborative relationships then the prospect of restructuring along lines antithetical to the interests of the professions produced the condition of 'unity through adversity'; a scenario which continues to be a significant stimulus for collaboration.

In this section, I will consider the role of the developments in allied health organization more explicitly by drawing on case-study data from a study of three different approaches to hospital organizational design (Boyce, 1996). The three models, and their closely related variants, represent the major classes of organizational design relevant to the allied health professions which are being implemented in Australia. Data were collected from interviews with 60 members of staff from medical, nursing, allied health and administrative backgrounds, observational strategies and an examination of documentary evidence. The case studies involved three acute-care Australian hospitals of approximately 600 beds. The different organizational models can only be briefly sketched here, but the key features were as follows.

Classical medical model. This model is the traditional Australian approach to allied health organization and is still the most numerous today. For the purposes of the research it acted as the reference model. In the classical medical model the professions are arranged as separate profession hierarchies with a profession manager appointed from the profession within a broader medical division structure. The profession managers are accountable for management of human and financial resources and report to an executive-level medical manager (salaried non-clinical role). The medical manager (medical director) acts as the allied health *and* the medical representative on top management committees.

Allied health division model. This model is the fastest growing approach to allied health organization in Australian hospitals. In an allied health division model the professions continue to be arranged as separate profession hierarchies with a profession manager appointed from the profession. The professions are organized as separate departments within an allied health division structure under the management of an allied health qualified director. The director is typically responsible for the management of human and financial resources of the division. The allied health division may exist as a stand-alone unit reporting to the chief executive officer of the hospital. Alternatively, it may exist as a division within a medical division structure, but the key feature is the separation of medical and allied health representation. In this arrangement the allied health director holds the function of representing the allied health professions on top management committees.

Unit dispersement model. This model of organization is often advocated by management consultants during restructuring exercises and by a significant proportion of health care executives. It is vigorously opposed by allied health profession associations and unions. The level of implementation of the model is low, with fewer than 10 examples known nationally. Despite its low implementation rate, the model is influential in thinking on the organizational design of hospitals because of its association with the concepts of decentralization and devolvement of authority to medical clinicians. In the unit dispersement model, allied health profession hierarchies are eliminated and individual/professionals or groups of professionals are directly employed by the constituent clinical units of the hospital under the direct management of a medical *clinician* manager.[54] Heads of each allied health discipline (profession leaders) are appointed but their role is restricted to advising on professional standards. Profession leaders have no managerial authority over the senior members of their discipline employed by the medical clinician managers of the clinical units. The representation of the allied health professions at the executive level is complex and is typically 'shared' between the medical clinician managers and sometimes an allied health representative selected on a rotational basis from the profession leaders. The dispersed and ambiguous nature of the allied health representative function is a key characteristic of this model of organization.

A central conclusion from the research was that local workplace organization can effect the influence and control exercized by the allied health professions depending on the structural conditions through which profession resources are managed. The research findings were consistent with many of those of Øvretveit (1988) about the under-recognized influence of workplace organization on the autonomy and independence of the British professions allied to medicine.

Where allied health professions have greater sovereignty over governance structures, their control over the nature of services provided can also be expected to be higher. Sovereignty over governance, as an expression of independence from medical management, also provides greater opportunities in institutional policy, planning and decision-making forums to advocate an allied health philosophy of care. When compared with the reference model, the classical medical model, the unit dispersement model was associated with greater formal involvement by medicine in the organization of the work of the allied health professions, whereas the allied health division model was associated with the least involvement.

Organizational designs such as the allied health division model and its variants are associated with greater profession management autonomy and organizational influence, and further, the unit dispersement model and its variants are more likely to be associated with a reduction in profession management autonomy and organizational influence in the managerial domain relative to the reference model. There was consistent evidence that the incorporation of a direct and legitimate (as contextually defined) representative of the allied health professions located in the top management strata of the hospital played a crucial role in communicating the importance of allied health objectives and their unique perspective on care.

An unambiguous direct representative position also played an important part in demonstrating that the institution could derive tangible organizational benefits from supporting collective forms of 'allied health' organization. Where the representation of allied health in top management forums was either ambiguous or mediated by a medical representative, hospital managers found it more difficult to articulate the benefits to the organization which accrued from the allied health professions aside from functions related to patient care.

Structural conditions affected the ease with which the professions could act as a unified 'power block' within the hospital. The unit dispersement model appeared to offer superior opportunities for influence by the allied health professions in the clinical domain and the managerial domain at the subunit level. The division of allied health model appeared to offer superior opportunities for influence at the organizational level through the visibility of the director of allied health position and its legitimacy as the organizationally endorsed 'voice' of allied health.

The nature of the structural framework in which interprofessional transactions were conducted was fundamentally important to the production of collaborative relationships *between* the allied health professions. A review of the literature reveals a lack of studies about how the allied health professions negotiate collectivity, cooperation and conflict in terms of interprofessional relations in organizational settings. Whilst there is some coverage in relation to the clinical domain, such as teamwork, very little is known about how managerial or strategic organizational issues are negotiated as a function of collective allied health behaviour. The received view has been that the allied health professions are inevitably rivalrous and have great difficulty working together (Beattie, 1995; Begun and Lippincott, 1993; Colman, 1992; du Toit, 1995; Gardner and McCoppin, 1995).

An organizational design which institutionalizes formal cooperative processes reinforces organizational expectations of collective rather than separatist behaviour amongst the individual professions. Wheeler and Grice (1996) and Boyce (1993a) have identified models of organization and cooperative processes whereby the tendency toward profession tribalism or separatism can be de-emphasized. However, a structural framework, although important in achieving this outcome, will not be sufficient without an investment in human and financial resources to support collective processes and meaningful participation.

The values which underpinned the philosophy of care associated with the allied health professions was typically referred to in the case-study sites as the 'allied health perspective'; a perspective which interviewees of all backgrounds recognized as qualitatively different from both the medical and the nursing perspectives. The institutionalization of an 'allied health perspective' into the norms of organizational decision-making and planning was a key mechanism in the reproduction of 'allied health' as an organizational entity. It was also the mechanism through which the allied health professions advocated their philosophy of care and sought to obtain an equitable share of resources to operationalize their care services.

Where the managerial elite of the organization perceived the 'allied health perspective' to be unified and contributing to organizational capabilities, the 'allied health perspective', and the collective processes which underpinned the perspective, were endorsed as valuable to the organization. The incorporation of the 'allied health perspective' into the norms of organizational life strengthens the claims of the allied health professions to greater independence and autonomy outside the supervisory management gaze of the medical profession.

The findings of the study also showed that senior non-medical hospital managers were under-recognized as important to the 'allied health' independence project. Non-medical managers are a focus for shaping the recognition of 'allied health' as contributing to organizational capabilities and competitive advantage (Chandler, 1992; Long and Vickers-Koch, 1995). This was most evident in the division of allied health model where the direct representatives of allied health penetrated the strategic-level decision-making apparatus of the hospital and achieved influence by shaping the perceptions of senior hospital managers on a routine basis.

In contrast, in the unit dispersement model it was medical clinician managers who shaped, filtered and interpreted the 'voice' of allied health in top-level forums to non-medical managers. Where medical clinician managers perceived the role of the allied health professions as primarily limited to a clinical resource operating at the subunit level there was great difficulty in the 'voice' of allied health being heard outside a clinically bound framework.

Organizational arrangements in which a collective 'allied health' grouping was supported in structural, resource and participation terms was more likely to evolve an 'allied health profession community' subculture. This is explained in part by the routinization of interprofessional social contact, favourable institutional conditions for shared-norm development and explicit organizational expectations of collective behaviour. The case-study research showed that the formation of an allied health subculture was greatest in the division of allied health model, followed by the classical medical model and the unit dispersement model.

The development of allied health as a 'profession community' suggested that the conventional understanding of 'allied health' as 'allied to medicine' could be undergoing a steady transformation in Australia to a phenomenon of 'allied to each other'. Subculture development was characterized by an increasingly apparent managerial and clinical interdependence, an emergent collective identity and a recognition within the cohort of profession managers that they were a network of peers rather than a set of competitors. The emergence of allied health as a 'profession community' in organizational arenas is influenced by structural and environmental conditions which may enhance or diminish the expression of subculture development.

The attainment of more autonomous management structures for health occupations has often been equated with an occupational strategy of professionalization through legitimizing the recognition of the institutional authority of the occupation (Alexander, 1984; Clinton and Nelson, 1995;

Porter, 1992; Wicks, 1995). Although organizational models which lead to outcomes such as increased profession management autonomy may be shown to reduce medical control and increase the institutional authority of the professions, this does not necessarily equate to a substantive change to the overall dominance of medicine.

An important caveat needs to be noted in relation to the importance of organizational arrangements. Greater sovereignty over management structures in hospitals can produce increased influence for the 'allied health perspective' and the underpinning allied health values and philosophy of care. This influence may translate into an impact on shaping clinical service offerings and corporate decision-making. However, it cannot be assumed that the care values of the allied health professions are especially client-centred or quarantined from the influence of the biomedical paradigm from which most of the disciplines have been derived.⁵⁵ The evidence from the case studies was, however, that the allied health perspective was perceived by other organizational actors as favouring a more holistic and preventive approach to health care than the medical perspective.

Managerialism and the subjugation of care and caring

The environment of change being faced by Australian allied health professions cannot be separated from the broader socio-political and economic changes in industrialized countries as they attempt to restructure fundamentally the nature of health care (Ham *et al.*, 1990). Irrespective of the philosophy underpinning the reforms, transformational change has been created in the 'business' of health care and in the social relations between the health professions and the agents of management.

At an organizational level the public hospital has been reconstructed from an institutional site of socially motivated service provision to a quasi-business enterprise in which economic rationalism, efficiency and effectiveness sit uncomfortably with principles of compassion, care, access and equity (Austin, 1989). The most stark image of this transition is reflected in the reconstruction of the 'patient' or 'client' to 'customer' (Gage, 1995; Scott, 1993). Also observable is the accompanying transition in the ethos of care to one in which consideration is given to the opportunity cost of treating particular kinds of customers according to their impact on the institutional bottom line (Boyce, 1994a; Duckett, 1994; Owens, 1995). In this scenario the patient is increasingly reduced to an accounting principle.

The introduction of devolved budgets and clinician management structures organized around the equivalent of clinical directorates, or what in the business world are recognizable as variants of strategic business units, has a profound impact on health professionals and the commodification of health care (Bartlett and Ghoshal, 1993; Boyce, 1994b). From the perspective of the health professions, the impact of change is one in which they are increasingly colonized into the managerialist framework in which care is subjugated to a concern for costs and the realities of doing business in a competitive industry.

Kendall's (1994) powerful insider account of the impact of economic rationalism following the implementation of a purchaser–provider model in New Zealand is illuminating. Productivity management, pruning of costs, performance monitoring, variation measuring and the construction of patients as 'secondary customers' are prominent in Kendall's account. Also prominent is the necessity of limiting the scope of the practitioner's treating and caring roles to activities consistent with a business ethos, such that the legitimacy of caring is suppressed in favour of treatments able to be costed:

> therapists who are multi-skilled must confine their practice to interventions that provide the outcome most valued by the frontline services [internal purchasers]. This paradigm of only providing what is most valued by customers is indeed a new mind set, but the reality that businesses operate under (Kendall 1994, p. 10).

This notion of health care, together with its fundamental underpinning ideology of managerialism and economic rationalism, is the site of contest about how the future of health care will be shaped (Hunter, 1994). The contested nature of health care challenges health professionals and organized professions to position themselves in terms of public advocacy within a broader charter of social responsibility. Equally importantly, the daily dilemma of reconciling a form of professionalism valued for its commercial efficiency and notions of care situated in responding to human need and frailty have to be confronted both by individual professionals and by their associations.

The problematic nature of professionalism and caring has been well described in the literature, particularly in relation to the nursing profession (Davies, 1995c; Witz, 1994). Davies (1995c, p. 149), for example, notes from her analysis of nursing that 'caring stands in a complex relation to scientific knowledge' and the basis of professionalism. The emergence of managerialism in its policy-relevant and operationally-focused forms stands in a new and potentially contradictory relation to both caring and professionalism. Harrison (1995) has demonstrated how the impact of managerialism and internal market reforms have challenged basic tenets of professionalism such as clinical autonomy.

The case study of Australian allied health professions demonstrates how they have responded at various levels to the challenge of health system reform to secure greater autonomy and participation in shaping change. A key strategy has been to organize under the umbrella of 'allied health' and to foster greater group identity and collective activity. It is possible within this movement to detect concerns of the professions about preserving their market position and protecting and extending the limited control they have established over procedural and knowledge bases relevant to their disciplines. At the same time, they aspire to advocate for their perspective on care and caring in top-level organizational and policy forums from which they had formerly been excluded or represented by medicine. Organization under the umbrella of 'allied health' has been shown to improve their chances of direct participation.

Conclusions

In this chapter I have argued that it is factors outside the clinical care domain, that is, organizational and managerial factors, which are of increasing importance to determining the power and autonomy of the health professions and the dominance of particular philosophical and operational approaches to 'care' in institutional settings.

Key issues impacting on all health professions are managerial accountability, responsible cost control over clinical services, continuity in patient care services across organizational settings and funding changes based on internal market reforms and clinical costing. At the institutional level the key changes have been the reform of organizational structures such that the sites of clinical care have been transformed into key operational subunits of strategic importance to resource management and organizational viability (Boyce, 1993b; Duckett, 1994; Harrison and Pollitt, 1994; Packwood *et al.*, 1991).

I have used the Australian allied health professions in this chapter as a case study of the profound nature of change occurring in the midst of reform of the health sector. The professions report both positive and negative effects on their power, autonomy and control over the context of care. A feature of change at the institutional level, and one that has been similarly observed in a study of British nursing (Witz, 1994), is the greater variability of the experiences of change.

The old ways, the stable ways, the systemwide ways are diminishing and local organizational experiences are likely to be different from those of neighbouring institutions. This is to be expected in a 'system' moving toward competitive market principles in which advantage is exploited and each player tries to manoeuvre within the market and develop a niche for their capabilities. Dealing with system variability rather than the more stable and predictable environment of the outcomes of central planning is one of the major challenges to the organized profession associations.

In the case of the Australian allied health professions I have traced the emergence of an 'allied health movement' at national, state and organizational levels. The evidence of more collaborative and cooperative organizational arrangements is suggestive of cultural change through the emergence of an 'allied health' subculture. There was also evidence that the development of an 'allied health perspective', rather than a raft of individual discipline views, can create more cooperative approaches to clinical relations and treatment protocols. Strickland (1995) and Wheeler and Grice (1996) have predicted similar outcomes within the Canadian and British therapy professions from more collaborative approaches. Wheeler and Grice's concept of an agency or bureau organizational model as a means of operationalizing the collaborative objective, although more limited in its scope, has similarities to the Australian concept of an allied health division model.

Cultural change achieved in new organizational approaches such as the allied health division model within Australian hospitals has been fundamental to driving changes at the national and state levels. Part of the cultural change emerging is the transition from an 'allied to medicine' construction of allied health to one of 'allied to each other'. This transition, if it is able to move beyond its current formative stage, is likely to impact further upon the relationship with medicine and require a less dependent interpretation of interprofessional relations than that which underpins medical dominance theories.

Endnotes

5.1 For a discussion of this point from the perspective of the United Kingdom, see Lorbiecki (1995).

5.2 The allied health director has much in common with a therapy services manager described in studies of the reorganization of health professions in the United Kingdom (Øvretveit, 1991, 1992). However, in the Australian context, the allied health director typically includes managerial responsibility for a more diverse set of services, and may include pharmacy, medical records and information management, medical librarians, prosthetics and orthodics, chaplaincy, special school services, biomedical engineering, clinical photography, optometry and dentists but rarely radiography or medical laboratory science. More recently, a number of allied health directors have been appointed at a regional level.

5.3 The author is the director of the National Allied Health Best Practice Consortium.

5.4 In a variant of this model, a shared governance arrangement may be in place between a medical clinician manager, a unit nurse executive and a unit business manager.

5.5 The social work profession must be considered somewhat of an exception within the 'allied health' rubric in this regard. See, for example, Bloor and Dawson (1994) who demonstrated that social workers exhibited more challenging behaviour to the dominant medical culture than other allied health professionals.

References

ABS 1991: *Characteristics of persons employed in health occupations, Australia (Catalogue no. 4346.0).* Canberra: Australian Bureau of Statistics.

Ackroyd, S. 1995: Nurses, management and morale: a diagnosis of decline in the NHS hospital service. In Soothill, K., Mackay, L. and Webb, C. (eds), *Interprofessional relations in health care.* London: Edward Arnold, 31–45.

Alexander, J. 1984: Organizational foundations of nursing roles: an empirical assessment. *Social Science and Medicine* **18**, 1045–52.

ANF 1991: *Health service organisational structures: policy statement and discussion paper.* North Fitzroy: Australian Nursing Federation.

APA 1994: *Position statement and discussion paper on hospital restructuring.* Melbourne: Australian Physiotherapy Association.

Austin, R.E. 1989: *The changing political economy of hospitals: the emergence of the 'business model' hospital.* Unpublished PhD thesis. Blacksburg, VA: Virginia Polytechnic Institute and State University.

Bartlett, C.A. and Ghoshal, S. 1993: Beyond the M-form: toward a managerial theory of the firm. *Strategic Management Journal* **14**, 23–46.

Beattie, A. 1995: War and peace among the health tribes. In Soothill, K., Mackay, L. and Webb, C. (eds), *Interprofessional relations in health care.* London: Edward Arnold, 11–30.

Begun, J.W. and Lippincott, R.C. 1993: *Strategic adaption in the health professions: meeting the challenges of change.* San Francisco, CA: Jossey-Bass.

Berry, M. 1994: Management of the therapy professions in the National Health Service of the 1990s. Unpublished Master's thesis. University of Kent, UK.

Blayney, K.D. and Fitz, P.A. 1990: The allied health professions: a critical resource in the future of health care. In *Perspectives on the health professions,* OP-2. Durham, NC: Pew Health Professions Programs, Duke University, 5–21.

Bloor, G. and Dawson, P. 1994: Understanding professional culture in organisation context. *Organisation Studies* **15**, 275–95.

Boyce, R.A. 1991: Hospital restructuring – the implications for allied health professions. *Australian Health Review* **14**, 147–54.

Boyce, R.A. 1992: New models of organisation in Australian hospitals and their implications for skill development in health professions. *Australian Communication Quarterly* (Summer), 9–11.

Boyce, R.A. 1993a: Internal market reforms of health care systems and the allied health professions: an international perspective. *International Journal of Health Planning and Management* **8**, 201–17.

Boyce, R.A. 1993b: The organisational design of hospitals – a critical review: a report on the 1992 Australian College of Health Service Executives Overseas Study Award, College monograph 1. North Ryde, NSW: Australian College of Health Service Executives.

Boyce, R.A. 1994a: Health industry reform in Australia: the implications of casemix funding. *QBiz (Queensland University of Technology)* 6–7.

Boyce, R.A. 1994b: Organisational design: patterns, policy and promises in hospital restructuring. *Australian Casemix Bulletin* **6**, 9–13.

Boyce, R.A. 1995: The business of economic reform of health care: what's allied health got to do with it? *Proceedings of the South West Pacific Region Dietitians Conference (Including the 14th National Conference of the Dietitians Association of Australia).* Brisbane: Dietitians Association of Australia.

Boyce, R.A. 1996: *The organisation of allied health professions in Australian general hospitals.* PhD thesis. Brisbane: Queensland University of Technology.

Bremner, J. 1993: Allied health working party report. *Medical Scientists Association of Victoria Annual Report.* Melbourne: Medical Scientists Association of Victoria, 6.

Bruhn, J.G. 1993: Shaping the future boundaries of occupational therapy. *Journal of Allied Health* **22**, 293–301.

Catchlove, B. 1991: Changing the management structure at the Royal Children's Hospital. *Australian Health Review* **14**, 86–8.

Chandler, A.D. 1992: Organizational capabilities and the economic history of the industrial enterprise. *Journal of Economic Perspectives* **6**, 79–100.

Clinton, M. and Nelson, S. 1995: Issues and trends in nurse management. In Clinton, M. and Scheiwe, D. (eds), *Management in the Australian health care industry*. Pymble: Harper Educational, 587–626.

Collins, D. 1993: The professional role of physiotherapists, the 1990 Act and the Patient's Charter. Unpublished Master's thesis. Swansea: University College Swansea.

Davies, C. 1995a: *Gender and the professional predicament in nursing*. Buckingham: Open University Press.

Davies, C. 1995b: Managing to care in the new NHS. In Davies, C. *Gender and the professional predicament in nursing*. Buckingham: Open University Press, 155–78.

Davies, C. 1995c: Professionalism and the condundrum of care. In Davies, C. *Gender and the professional predicament in nursing*. Buckingham: Open University Press, 133–54.

Duckett, S.J. 1994: Hospital and departmental management in the era of accountability: addressing the new management challenges. *Australian Health Review;* **17**, 116–31.

Duckett, S.J., Scarf, C.G., Schmiede, A.M. and Weaver, C.J. 1981: *The organisation of medical staff in Australian hospitals*. Melbourne: Longman Cheshire.

du Toit, D. 1995: The allied health professions in Australia: physio, occupational and speech therapy professions. In Lupton, G.M. and Najman, J.M. (eds), *Sociology of health and illness: Australian readings*. 2nd edn. South Melbourne: Macmillan Education Australia, 276–97.

Flynn, R. 1992: Medical autonomy and managerial encroachment. In Flynn, R. (ed.), *Structures of control in health management*. London: Routledge, 23–54.

Furnham, A., Pendleton, D., Manicom, C. 1981: The perception of different occupations within the medical profession. *Social Science and Medicine* **15E**, 289–300.

Gage, M. 1995: Re-engineering of health care: opportunity or threat for occupational therapists. *Canadian Journal of Occupational Therapy* **62**, 197–207.

Gardner, H. and McCoppin, B. 1995: Struggle for survival by health therapists, nurses and medical scientists. In Gardner, H. (ed.), *The politics of health: the Australian experience*. 2nd edn. Melbourne: Churchill Livingstone, 371–427.

Giaimo, S. 1995: Health care reform in Britain and Germany: recasting the political bargain with the medical profession. *Governance* **8**, 354–79.

Hafferty, F.W. and McKinlay, J.B. (eds) 1993: *The changing medical profession*. New York: Oxford University Press.

Ham, C., Robinson, R. and Benzeval, M. 1990: *Health check: health care reforms in an international context*. London: King's Fund Institute.

Harrison, S. 1995: Clinical autonomy and planned markets: the British case. In Saltman, R.B., von Otter, C. (eds), *Implementing planned markets in health care: balancing social and economic responsibility*. Buckingham: Open University Press, 156–76.

Harrison, S. and Pollitt, C. 1994: *Controlling health professionals: the future of work and organization in the National Health Service*. State of Health Series. Buckingham: Open University Press.

Hickson, D.J., Hinings, C.R., Lee, C.A., Schneck, R.E. and Pennings, J.M. 1971: A strategic contingencies theory of intraorganizational power. *Administrative Science Quarterly* **16**, 216–29.

Hugman, R. 1991a: Organization and professionalism: the social work agenda in the 1990s. *British Journal of Social Work* **21**, 199–216.

Hugman, R. 1991b: *Power in caring professions.* London: Macmillan Education.

Hugman, R. 1995: Contested territory and community services: interprofessional boundaries in health and social care. In Soothill, K., Mackay, L. and Webb, C. (eds), *Interprofessional relations in health care.* London: Edward Arnold, 31–45.

Hunter, D.J. 1994: From tribalism to corporatism: the managerial challenge to medical dominance. In Gabe, J., Kelleher, D. and Williams, G. (eds), *Challenging medicine.* London: Routledge, 1–22.

Institute of Medicine 1989: *Allied health services: avoiding crises.* Washington, DC: National Academy Press.

Irvine, R. and Graham, J. 1994: Deconstructing the concept of profession: a prerequisite to carving a niche in a changing world. *Australian Occupational Therapy Journal* **41**, 9–18.

Keen, J. and Malby, R. 1992: Nursing power and practice in the United Kingdom National Health Service. *Journal of Advanced Nursing* **17**, 863–70.

Kendall, S. 1994: The New Zealand health reforms: impacts on one occupational therapy service. *New Zealand Journal of Occupational Therapy* **45**, 8–11.

Larkin, G.V. 1988: Medical dominance in Britain: image and historical reality. *Milbank Quarterly* **66** (supplement 2), 117–32.

Lloyd-Smith, W. 1995: NHS trusts, the market and occupational therapy. *British Journal of Therapy and Rehabilitation* (September), 473–77.

Long, C. and Vickers-Koch, M. 1995: Using core capabilities to create competitive advantage. *Organisational Dynamics* (Summer), 7–22.

Lorbiecki, A. 1995: Clinicians as managers: convergence or collision? In Soothill, K., Mackay, L. and Webb, C. (eds), *Interprofessional relations in health care.* London: Edward Arnold, 88–106.

Macklin, J. 1992: Allied health and the National Health Strategy. *The First National Allied Health Services Conference: Unity Through Diversity.* Proceedings on audiotape. Melbourne: Austin Hospital.

NAHMGWP 1993: *Discussion paper: the development of a national allied health management association.* Convenor T. Aslett, Austin Hospital, Melbourne: National Allied Health Management Group Working Party.

NHSU 1991a: *The Australian health jigsaw: integration of health care delivery.* National Health Strategy Unit Issues Paper 1. Melbourne: National Health Strategy Unit.

NHSU 1993: *Health that works: reform and best practice in the Australian health industry.* National Health Strategy Unit Issues Paper 7. Melbourne: National Health Strategy Unit.

Øvretveit, J.A. 1988: *Professional power and the state: a study of five professions in state welfare agencies in the UK.* Unpublished PhD thesis. Uxbridge, Middlesex: Brunel University.

Øvretveit, J.A. 1991: Future organisation of therapy services. *Health Services Management* **87**, 78–80.

Øvretveit, J.A. 1992: *Therapy services: organisation, management and autonomy.* Chur: Harwood Academic Publishers.

Øvretveit, J.A. 1994: Physiotherapy service contracts and 'business autonomy'. *Physiotherapy* **80**, 372–6.

Owens, H. 1995: Paying for health care through casemix. In Gardner, H. (ed.), *The politics of health: the Australian experience.* 2nd edn. Melbourne: Churchill Livingstone, 284–305.

Packwood, T., Keen, J. and Buxton, M. 1991: *Hospitals in transition: the resource management experiment.* Buckingham: Open University Press.

Porter, S. 1992: The poverty of professionalisation: a critical analysis of strategies for the occupational advancement of nursing. *Journal of Advanced Nursing* 17, 720–8.

PSA 1990: *Allied health departments in public hospitals.* Sydney: Public Service Association.

Robb, J.H. 1975: Power, profession and administration: an aspect of change in English hospitals. *Social Science and Medicine* 9, 373–82.

Robinson, J., Gray, A. and Elkan, R. (eds) 1992: *Policy issues in nursing.* Buckingham: Open University Press.

Sachs, D. and Labovitz, D.R. 1994: The caring occupational therapist: scope of professional roles and boundaries. *The American Journal of Occupational Therapy* 48, 997–1005.

Safriet, B.J. 1994: Impediments to progress in health care workforce policy: license and practice laws. *Inquiry* 31: 310–17.

Saltman, R.B. and von Otter, C. 1995: *Implementing planned markets in health care: balancing social and economic responsibility.* Buckingham: Open University Press.

Scarf, C.J. 1991: Clinical management structure: the Royal Prince Alfred Hospital experience. *Australian Health Review* 14, 83–5.

Schemm, R.L. 1993: Bridging conflicting ideologies: the origins of American and British occupational therapy. *The American Journal of Occupational Therapy* 48, 1082–88.

Scott, W.R. 1993: The organization of medical care services: towards an integrated theoretical model. *Medical Care Review* 50, 271–302.

Strickland, A. 1995: Collaborating to create important strategic partnerships for occupational therapy. *Canadian Journal of Occupational Therapy* 62, 237–41.

Weeks, G.R. 1991: The allied health movement and changing organisational structures in hospitals: a pharmacy perspective. *Australian Journal of Hospital Pharmacy* 21, 359–67.

Wheeler, N. and Grice, D. 1996: Generic or specialist: a model for contracting the professions. *British Journal of Therapy and Rehabilitation* 3, 11–15.

Wicks, D. 1995: Nurses and doctors and discourses of healing. *Australian and New Zealand Journal of Sociology* 31, 122–39.

Witz, A. 1994: The challenge of nursing. In Gabe, J., Kelleher, D. and Williams, G. (eds), *Challenging medicine.* London: Routledge, 23–45.

Young, A.P. 1995: The politics of professional power in today's health-care market. *British Journal of Therapy and Rehabilitation* 2, 562–5.

Part 3: Exploration of 'non-Western' views of care

Editors' introduction

It is hardly news to suggest that 'non-Western' views of care have been neglected in the West. This ignoring of global diversity is curious, for visits to the Indian subcontinent in the late 1960s by pop stars, such as the Beatles, seeking spiritual guidance and inspiration produced a rather unexpected focus by the young on an alternative set of approaches to and understandings of the human condition. However, much less evident around that time was any interest espoused by those in positions of power and authority within Western democracies in 'non-Western' views about anything. However, the phrase 'non-Western' produces the rub. Whereas 'Western' views can be identified with some coherence, the range and diversity of the possible alternatives are enormous. In brief, 'non-Western' is a negative definition which suggests that one can draw together all that is not directly Western-influenced. That this is both naive and mistaken is illustrated by our two contributions which highlight quite distinct approaches working within two very different contexts.

Developing interest in the late 1980s and 1990s in 'non-Western' cultural values among those involved with administering health and social services in Western countries came about not so much in terms of what alternative approaches had to offer but in response to a growing recognition that groups in society, particularly minority ethnics, were disadvantaged in a variety of ways. Azmi argues powerfully that 'The implications of social diversity for the provision of social care are significant and far-reaching' (p. 102). His particular contribution begins to tackle the important question of how the recognition of social diversity impacts upon contemporary notions of professionalism. Azmi examines the welfare situation of the Muslim minority community in metropolitan Toronto in Canada and in so doing is, in fact, focusing on an increasingly usual circumstance in the contemporary world. We need to recognize that radically different communities are living, either easily or uneasily, near or next to each other. Azmi points to the effect of occupational professionalism which increasingly demands specialization and a focus on segregated realms of human activity. Nevertheless, he argues that all health and social care professionals must realize that their work represents a specific ideological viewpoint which may be radically at odds with the ideological viewpoint of the sometimes diverse communities being served. Perhaps more dangerously, the idea of secular and specialized types of care being administered through professional occupational forms is thought to give the contemporary health and social care occupations universal validity. While Azmi recognizes that the idea of a transcendent form of care may be an alluring notion, his own evidence suggests that such a belief represents a grand illusion.

If further evidence is needed to challenge such a notion, Fernandes and Mazumdar focus on the multifaceted Indian cultural and economic contexts, considering the suitability of the Western model of social work to what they describe as 'the constantly metamorphosing Indian social realities' (p. 138). While the profession of social work was largely derived from the US model, it increasingly came to be recognized as inappropriate. Important paradigm shifts came in the late 1970s. Fernandes and Mazumdar note how several Indian social work educators – trained in the United States and later teaching and practising in India – began to realize the significance of the cultural variants in social work practice. They emphasized the need to incorporate Indian thought and as well as traditions of work and perceptions of needs to indigenize social work practice and education.

Both contributions make a point perhaps more easily said but less easily applied. As Fernandes and Mazumdar stress, 'There is a need for the social worker to be able to think and reflect on the cultural situation before determining the best course of action to help clients, instead of mechanically and routinely applying techniques taken from the West'. In a world where media communicators talk glibly of a 'global village', we do need, as Azmi emphasizes, to consider 'the implications of social diversity for the provision of social care'.

6

Professionalism and social diversity

Shaheen Azmi

Introduction

The implications of social diversity for the provision of social care are significant and far-reaching. Although these have been explored from a multitude of perspectives little work has been done in exploring how the recognition of social diversity impacts upon contemporary notions of professionalism. This chapter will explore this issue with reference to qualitative research conducted into the welfare situation of the Muslim minority community in metropolitan Toronto, Canada (Azmi, 1996). This research detailed perceptions regarding the welfare response to wife abuse in the Muslim community, both of welfare workers from mainstream welfare institutions and from within the community itself. Divergent perceptions that emerged from this context were related to distinctive and competing ideological outlooks regarding welfare conception and welfare provision. That situations of welfare provision in contexts of social diversity may be complicated by the presence of competing welfare ideologies is identified as having fundamental implications for social care professions. The primary implication to be explored is that social care professionals must acknowledge fundamental boundaries to the extension of their professional work in many contexts of social diversity.

Although the health and social care professions share some structural features, each of these professions has a unique history and retains many distinguishing characteristics. For purposes of clarity it is therefore valuable to specify a specific branch of the health and social care professions for review. In this chapter social work will be focused on, partially because of my own familiarity with it, but also because of all the social care occupations none has made a more self-conscious effort to develop itself according to a professional ideal than has social work (Lubove, 1965).

Professionalism in the provision of social care has recently been reviewed from various critical perspectives. For example, prominent works such as those of Wilding (1982) and Hugman (1991) have focused on the idea of 'social power' as being a central concept explaining the origins and operation of professionalism in social care provision. The approach of social diversity outlined in this chapter will offer another critical perspective, which in many ways is complementary to the perspective offered by the concept of social power. This approach will locate social care professionalism in a broader context and will highlight the possibility of competing viewpoints regarding occupational norms in the provision of social care. It will be contended that social care professionals must acknowledge this possibility in their work if they are to operate adequately and with integrity in a diverse society and world.

Research in the Muslim community of Toronto

The research in the context of the Muslim community of metropolitan Toronto consisted of 18 qualitative semi-structured interviews conducted with individuals who were in some way involved in the welfare response to wife abuse in the Muslim community. Respondents included Muslim and non-Muslim individuals working in a variety of contexts. The list of respondents included individuals involved in religious and community institutions within the Muslim community, and individuals active in ethnic community or mainstream health and social care institutions.

The problem of wife abuse in the Muslim community was chosen to focus research on the basis that it was a situation which compelled interaction between individuals from the two communities. It promised the best situation to picture how individuals from both the Muslim community and from mainstream institutions understood the nature of their own work and that of others working to address the same concern. Of course, the situation was complicated by overlaps – by the fact that some individuals from within the Muslim community were active in mainstream institutions.

Research findings: competing ideologies of welfare

The research uncovered a situation where multiple ideologies of welfare and welfare response were present and related to competitive behaviour between sections of the Muslim community and the mainstream social welfare system. These multiple ideologies were classified in to two basic types, one an Islamic religious ideology and the other a secular liberal ideology. Each of these ideologies related to highly distinct perceptions regarding basic welfare phenomena, including distinct conception of definition and causation of wife abuse and the evaluation of its presence in the Muslim community and society in general. Correspondingly, distinct perspectives on the appropriate responses to the problem were identified in terms of the appropriate social agents to respond to it and in terms of the appropriate characteristics and qualifications individual agents involved in this response should possess.

The Islamic religious ideology, as was to be expected, was espoused most clearly by individuals active in religious sectors of the Muslim community, but extended in varying degrees to some Muslim respondents active within other institutions including mainstream health and social care agencies. The secular liberal ideology was espoused most clearly by non-Muslim respondents active within mainstream institutions but extended in varying degrees to some Muslim respondents active in secular ethnic-based sectors within the Muslim community.

Ideological viewpoints on ideal traits for welfare agents

One realm within which the research found considerable difference between the Islamic and the secular liberal ideologies of welfare concerned their understanding of the ideal traits which should characterize agents active in the welfare response to wife abuse. Overall, respondents identified five qualities as being important factors in determining the effectiveness of welfare workers. These five factors included: beliefs and values, cultural sensitivity, technical knowledge and skill, position and authority, and personal sensitivity. Although respondents classified into both ideological groupings identified all of these five factors, they did so with differing patterns of emphasis and with clearly distinctive outlooks with regard to each.

Values and beliefs were the single most important category of importance to respondents who were classified in the Islamic ideological group. These respondents identified the religious beliefs and values maintained by welfare agents to be of great importance to the effectiveness of their work. For most of these respondents religious values and beliefs were the primary quality determining the suitability of welfare agents. In contrast, respondents who were classified in the secular liberal ideological group did not consider religious values or beliefs to be significant at all. A handful of these respondents did connect the effectiveness of welfare workers to the maintenance of progressive values, but most implied that the personal values and beliefs of welfare workers was irrelevant to welfare activity, the indication being that professional or occupational values superseded any effect of these personal values and beliefs.

Whereas respondents from the Islamic ideological group tended to emphasize values and beliefs as being the primary factor determining the effectiveness of welfare workers, respondents from the other ideological group primarily emphasized the two factors of cultural sensitivity and specialized knowledge and skill. Almost all of these respondents deemed both of these two factors to be critical and primary for the effectiveness of welfare workers responding to wife abuse. In contrast, most respondents from the Islamic ideological group did not consider either of these factors to be very significant. Some of these respondents instead emphasized the importance of religious knowledge *per se* and regarded religious knowledge concerning the problem being addressed as secondary.

The difference between the emphasis on specialized knowledge on the one hand and on religious knowledge on the other hand was reflected in the specific goals the two ideological groups identified as being the primary aims which should govern the welfare response to wife abuse. Respondents from the Islamic ideological group specified two interrelated primary goals. These were the saving of souls and the preservation of the family. These two goals were seen as interrelated because the second goal was seen by the respondents who identified it as being vital for the broader task of the saving of souls. Since the primary goal was the saving of souls, it was religious knowledge which was deemed the most important for the task at hand. In contrast, the primary goal formulated by most respondents from the other ideological group was that of the safety of women in abusive situations. Notably, the focus from this perspective was typically liberal and secular, the focus being clearly on the individual's immediate concerns rather than on other-worldly concerns or on family or group concerns associated with these. Since the primary aim identified was the remedying of a specific and immediate problem confronting an individual, it was specialized knowledge about the situation and marital interaction in general which was deemed the most important for the task at hand.

The outlook on the ideal welfare agent from the perspective of respondents expressing the Islamic welfare ideology was that of a religiously committed welfare worker whose activities would be governed primarily by religious goals and norms established within the religious tradition. In contrast, the outlook of the other ideological group was that of a secular welfare worker, whose goals and norms would be governed in reference to specialized knowledge and skill and to civic culture and legal codes.

Boundaries for welfare activity

Differences between the two identified conceptions were also apparent in reference to the identification of boundaries for welfare activity. Those who idealized the notion of a secular liberal welfare worker did not postulate any cultural or religious boundaries that by necessity would inhibit the activities of welfare workers. Since the emphasis was on individual care mediated by specialized knowledge and skill, which included some sense of cultural familiarity, the idea of a cultural or religious boundary was not envisioned. In contrast, those who idealized the concept of a religiously-committed welfare worker postulated a number of boundaries between welfare workers and service communities. For example, some respondents from this perspective indicated that only religiously committed welfare workers were capable of any effective work at all. These individuals implied a boundary of legitimacy between all service communities and all non-religiously-committed welfare workers. Other respondents advanced a less radical position indicating that only religiously-committed welfare workers were capable of effective work with their own religious communities. This view implied a boundary for welfare workers dictated by their own personal religious commitments.

In summary, significant sections of the Muslim community in Toronto clearly maintain ideological conceptions of welfare and care which are significantly at odds with Canadian mainstream welfare conceptions. Islamic ideology of welfare is integrated into a traditional Islamic religious world-view, which almost indistinguishably fuses realms of religion and welfare. It tends to give primary importance to religious identity and tends to divide the welfare world in relationship to it. The ideal welfare agent from this perspective is not only the one whose activities correspond with the traditional religious world-view but also the one whose being and character is primarily identified with it and the community of belief established around it. Correspondingly, the Islamic ideology of welfare envisions a boundary between the community of belief and all other communities. Notably, welfare activity beyond this boundary, if engaged in, is understood primarily as missionary in character.

In contrast Canadian mainstream ideology of welfare is essentially secular, strictly dividing between realms of religion and welfare, and is liberal in character in that it gives primary importance to individual rights above other considerations. This ideology tends to give primary importance to human identity in this world and does not in principle sanction the division of the welfare world along religious or other group lines. The ideal welfare agent from this perspective is the one who is primarily endowed with the specialized expertise to deal with the specific problem, any other identification of the agent with the client being secondary. Correspondingly, Canadian mainstream ideology of welfare does not envision boundaries of any fundamental character between communities within the human family.

Implications of ideological distinctions

The research findings outlined above offer compelling evidence of the vitality of multiple welfare ideologies corresponding to various forms of social diversity. The realities of social diversity cannot be contained into realms identified by arbitrary mental categories such as culture, ethnicity, race and the like, as social work writers on the area have almost uniformly conceived. Diversity in many cases, and certainly in the case of traditional religious civilizations such as Islam, corresponds to deeply entrenched religiously-centred world-views. These world-views inform understanding of all phenomena, including those activities categorized by modern health and social care professions as being in the realm of welfare (Azmi, 1992).

Professionalism and diversity in social work literature

The possibility that fundamental ideas of welfare are often contested notions in welfare activity in contexts of social diversity has not received much attention by social workers or other welfare professionals. It has been assumed that welfare as understood by the modern welfare professions are uncontested notions which are universally valid and which consequently can be legitimately applied upon all cultures. Even social work literature critically appraising social work professionalism in contexts of diversity makes such assumptions.

For example, Midgley's book (1981) entitled *Professional imperialism: social work in the Third World* represents the only substantial critical approach to social work professionalism advanced from the viewpoint of issues of diversity. A review of Midgley's main contentions would indicate that he too ignores the possibility that cultural distinctions may relate to fundamental ideological distinctions regarding the way welfare is understood.

Midgley advances the idea that social work in the Third World can be characterized as an example of 'professional imperialism'. He develops this critique of international social work upon his contention that the social work profession has been shaped by its roots in nineteenth century Western liberal culture. He details the history of social work in the European and US contexts and illustrates the profound imprint of liberal ideas and norms upon professional social work values. In particular he identifies the parochially liberal foundations of social work's professed fundamental value of individual self-determination. Midgley proceeds to detail how professional social work has been exported unthinkingly to cultures which do not share liberal values and beliefs. He argues that social work professionalism in these contexts has been inappropriate and even counter-productive to the social development of these cultures.

In response to what he formulates as professional imperialism, Midgley calls for the development of localized social work practices whose professional norms are structured around indigenous cultural characteristics and pragmatic social needs. He recognizes that there would be entrenched opposition to this idea, but he affirms the possibility in principle that new appropriate forms of social work can be identified which allow social work to 'retain its basic characteristics and commitments' but which effectively end the phenomenon of professional imperialism (p. 173). For Midgley, then, professional imperialism is not fundamental but is an unfortunate and reversible aspect of social work exportation to non-Western societies. From his perspective, professional social work is still an activity which is fundamentally portable across international borders of cultural diversity.

Midgley's fixation on 'cultural diversity' reflects a similar fixation among most welfare professionals towards defining problems of diversity almost exclusively within parochial 'cultural' or 'ethnic' categories. This fixation has the effect of obscuring the reality of ideological distinctions associated with cultural variation. The research reviewed above indicated that religious and cultural distinctions may conceal ideological distinctions, which in turn may vitally influence perceptions of welfare and welfare-related behaviour. In this context the implication is that Midgley's formulation of professional imperialism is inadequate.

Limitations in Midgley's concept of professional imperialism

Midgley's approach can be faulted for not recognizing sufficiently the possibility that indigenous ideological conceptions of welfare and welfare provision systems may exist in many societies to which modern social work has been exported. Undoubtedly, intensifying forces of modernization have undermined the vitality of these conceptions, and certainly they have eroded their corresponding welfare provision systems. However, the example of the Muslim minority community in Toronto would suggest that they have not completely disappeared even in minority contexts in Western societies.

Midgley, like most contemporary observers, does not recognize indigenous welfare ideologies and provision systems because they are not made in the image of modern secularized notions of welfare. Many cultures to which modern welfare professions have been extended, at least in the Muslim world and likely beyond, are rooted in non-secular traditional religious world-views. It is likely that these indigenous conceptions of welfare and their various provision systems are centred in traditional religious expressions in a manner analogous to that found among sections of the Muslim community in Toronto.

The implication of coherent indigenous ideologies of welfare associated with traditional religious world-views is significant. It would suggest that Midgley's formulation of the limitations of professional social work is not sufficiently fundamental. Midgley focused his entire analysis on the cultural limitations of professional social work's values and largely ignored the more fundamental ideological assumptions associated with its epistemological foundations. Having not recognized ideological variation to welfare conception, Midgley does not recognize the parochial character of professional social work's ideological assumptions. It is the parochial character of social work's ideological foundations which clearly imply more fundamental barriers to professional social work's portability than those acknowledged by Midgley.

Midgley's proposed solution to professional imperialism is a pragmatic social work, developed according to the contingencies and indigenous forces found in specific international settings. However, this solution does not sufficiently acknowledge that social work itself, in any recognizable form, that is, as a specialized profession, may not conform to the occupational norms of competing welfare ideologies. Correspondingly, the nature of social work's professional imperialism would appear to be much more fundamental than Midgley's formulation implies. Social work faces in social diversity ideological forms which may be completely hostile to its own form. The professional imperialism of social work in contexts of social diversity needs to be reformulated to reflect ideological realities.

Historical ideologies of professionalism and modern social work

Before proceeding to reformulate the idea of professional imperialism it is worthwhile to approach the parochial character of professional social work from another more theoretical angle, because it is this idea which is critical to understanding the truly profound character of social work's professional imperialism, and it is also this idea which is most deeply resisted by professional social workers.

Professional social work is not only parochial because it is deeply imbued with liberal values, as Midgley formulates, but it is more essentially parochial because it corresponds only to the ideological norms of modern notions of welfare and to the wider ideological norms of the modern world-view. To recognize that professional social work is essentially an expression of the welfare ideology of the modern world-view, it is sufficient to recognize that the very idea of a specialized profession, in its contemporary sense, is peculiar to the occupational norms of contemporary Western civilization, which is established on the foundations of the modern world-view.

Most sociological writing on professionalism implicitly acknowledges that the contemporary occupational form of 'professionalism' is characteristic only of notions of occupational organization associated with the modern outlook (Halmos, 1973; Vollmer and Mills, 1966). Blumer (1966, p. xi), for one, connects the two in writing:

> There is ample evidence for believing that modern society has a distinctive character which sets it apart from earlier societies. It is massive in scope, highly heterogeneous in composition, endowed with intrinsic pressures toward transformation, and confronted with an ever shifting world to which it has to adjust. It may be viewed quite validly as struggling for structure. One of the most interesting, important, and ill-understood aspects of this structuring process is the growth of professionalization.

There is a profound interconnection between any occupational form and the widest theoretical assumptions of the society it is established in. Modern professionalism has confused many to this simple truth because of the exaggerated importance given to some superficial traits retained from earlier stages of the development of professionalism in Western history. For example, modern professionalism retains some ideals of service and self-regulation which appear to be out of place in the context of modern liberal and bureaucratic forms of organization. However, the peculiarly modern character of the contemporary notion of professionalism is evident when the essential character of modern professionalism is exposed in relationship to its historical antecedents. The term 'profession' has been continuously employed for centuries to designate certain high-status occupations but its essential characteristics have changed in fundamental ways. A review of the history of professionalism would show that the term has been designated on the basis of radically distinct social characteristics over different historical periods. I will review some aspects of the history of professionalism in the English context to further illustrate the parochial character of modern professionalism.

The choice to review the history of the notion of professionalism in the English context was also made because it exposes alternate historical visions of occupational organization which, as will be displayed later with reference to the Muslim community context in Toronto, are very much still vital forms in today's diverse world.

Professionalism in historical context

The term 'profession' indicates the roots of the idea of professionalism in religious expression. One perspective from which to approach the history of the notion of professionalism is to trace the secularization of what was a traditional religious mode of occupational organization. Associated with this secularization was the elimination of the Church's monopoly in controlling various high-status classical occupations, including occupations in law, politics, the military and, most significant for our purposes, in the provision of welfare. The removal of the Church's monopoly was also associated with the gradual marginalization of religious-centred theoretical knowledge and the growing ascendance of rationalistic and scientific modes of knowledge as the basic epistemological foundations of these professions.

Regarding the history of the professions in England, Elliott (1972) identifies three major stages in the transformation of the notion of the professional ideal. These stages are associated with three historic periods in English history: the Middle Ages, the post-Reformation period, and the post-Industrial-Revolution modern period.

Religious professionalism: professionalism in the Middle Ages

In the Middle Ages the idea of a profession was intricately associated with religion as an idea and the Church as a social institution. The professions were just another expression of the religious ideals of the Church. As Rashdall (1936) writes, 'in the north of Europe the Church was simply a synonym for the professions' (p. 446).

Professionalism in the medieval sense was primarily an extension of religious life. It represented a means towards spiritual salvation by fulfilling a required service. It was not seen primarily as work but as a calling and was indistinguishable from the work of the Church. The highest of professions was the priesthood, and other occupations emulated its religious content and its formal characteristics. For example, welfare activity in the Middle Ages was primarily conducted in the context of Church-related institutions. There was no essential separation understood between the realms of religion and the realms of health or social care. The focus for all realms was the 'cure of souls' (McNeill, 1952), and all were entrusted to the supervision of the Church. As Kemp (1947, p. 36) writes:

> About the tenth century many parish churches, as well as cathedrals and monasteries, maintained hospitals as well as orphanages and institutions for the care of paupers. Even lepers were cared for. Special orders and brotherhoods developed, such as the Knights of St. John whose chief reason for being was to care for those who were sick or otherwise needed help.

The Church played a ubiquitous role in controlling access to most types of knowledge and education, including specialized education associated with the realms of health and social care. As Elliott (1972, p. 17) writes of the Church's role in the age:

> The universities were not directly clerical foundations, but most of their members had some links with the Church. Distinction at the university was an accepted route to position in the Church. Theology had pride of place in the curriculum as the 'queen of science'.

Education of prospective professionals in universities consisted primarily of religion-centred knowledge and abstract intellectual development. Specialized training and knowledge in some realms, such as medicine and law, were developed to some degree. However, specialized education was considered secondary to religious education and moral training, because these were deemed to be the most essential requirements for professional activity and life.

Status professionalism: professionalism after the Reformation

If religion was the overriding factor influencing the form assumed by professionalism in the Middle Ages, social status was the overriding factor influencing its developing form in the post-Reformation period. The growing power of secular authority in the form of a landed aristocracy supported the development of professionalism separate from religion and Church institutions.

Professional ideology which was entirely religion-centred was confronted with a competing secular ideology which idealized in its place the norms of the landed gentry. The emerging professional ideology was influenced by the ideal of the gentlemanly lifestyle associated with the aristocracy. Such a life was to follow a leisurely style, independent of the need to engage in manual labour or in trade or commerce. The professions in the fields of law, health care and the military were envisioned as extensions of the gentlemanly ideal. As Elliott (1972, p. 21) writes, 'The ideology of professionalism at this time stressed the independence of the professional from employer, client, economic pressure, even from work itself'. The performance of the specialized function of a professional was considered secondary to the primary ability to live a suitably leisured and cultured lifestyle. Being a professional represented more a confirmation of a status position than confirmation of practical expertise.

Correspondingly, specialized knowledge and expertise were not primary criteria defining professionalism. As Elliott writes (p. 32) 'Professional learning was not a specific and useful expertise so much as an acquaintance with a culture which had an accepted value in society, if no obvious vocational relevance'. Professional education even in centres such as Oxford and Cambridge aimed more at confirming refined culture and lifestyle than at fostering specialized knowledge and skill. The focus on theological education was replaced by greater attention to general classical learning. Specialized learning even in health care was marginal to the practice of the professional. As Elliott (p. 28) points out about a physician in the age of status professionalism:

> He might have extensive learning in classic literature and culture, but he depended on his gentlemanly manner, impressive behaviour and his clients' ignorance to develop a medical practice. In so far as a system of medical education existed at all by the end of the eighteenth century, it depended on the personal initiative of the aspirant to gain his medical knowledge.

The monopoly of Church institutions in controlling professional activity having ended, secular professional associations began to develop. In regard to health care, professional medical associations were inaugurated in the sixteenth century. Corresponding with the overall vision of status-based professionalism, membership in the professional associations was not based on educational qualification or specialized knowledge or skill but was rather based on whether prospective members had the latent status characteristics necessary for professional life.

Occupational professionalism: professionalism in the modern age

The overriding factor shaping the form of professionalism after the Industrial Revolution has been the rising notion of labour power as a commodity in an exchange economy and the association of status with occupation. The growth of capitalist thinking infused itself into status professionalism to create what is now the dominant contemporary understanding of the professionals as specialized self-regulated occupations. Specialized work was only a secondary aspect defining the professional in the cases of both spiritual and status professionalism. However, in the case of modern occupational notions of professionalism specialized work has emerged as the defining quality. In the modern period it is occupational expertise which confirms professional status and which accords the professions high status in society.

Corresponding to the emerging importance of occupation to professionalism has been the growing significance accorded to specialized and scientific knowledge as the theoretical foundations necessary for professional life. Consequently, it is the cultivation of practical expertise in a specialized activity which has become the primary focus of professional learning. Although moral and ethical considerations are still factors for the professional ideal they have increasingly been marginalized as requisite concerns for professional learning.

The intensified focus on specialized knowledge and education was reflected in the establishment in the nineteenth century of written examinations and specialized educational qualifications as the primary criteria for membership in professional associations. Intensified specialization of knowledge is also to be related to the enormous diversification of professional occupations since the nineteenth century. For example, the many new professions which have emerged since the nineteenth century in the realm of health and social care have reflected this specialization, including social work.

It is significant to note that occupational professionalism completes the process of secularization begun with status professionalism. During the period of status professionalism, the interconnections between the Church and the aristocracy were significant enough to insure that religion remained a significant force shaping the nature of professions and professional activity. Moreover, the priesthood was still understood to be the ideal and most prestigious profession in the hierarchy of professions. However, with occupational professionalism, the position of the Church as regulator, mediator and chief patron of professionals has been all but replaced by the secular state. The position of theological and religious learning as the main theoretical foundations for professionalism has been completely replaced by scientific learning. The position of the priesthood as the highest-status profession has been replaced by that of the physician. Indeed, secularization has proceeded to such a degree that even the priesthood itself has been forced to conform to secularized norms (Goldner *et al.*, 1973).

Ideologies of professionalism in the contemporary world

The historical development of the idea of professionalism indicates that the notion has fundamentally varied according to the overall world-view within which its norms have been defined. Professionalism has always been a form of occupational organization associated with a range of high-status primarily non-manual activities. However, the content of professionalism, its theoretical underpinnings, its norms and its institutional character have varied according to the world within which the idea has been operationalized.

It is significant to note that the historical periods of the idea of professionalism identified in the context of England relate to contemporary notions of professionalism evident in different cultural contexts today. In today's diversified world significant cultures retain world-views very similar in form to those identified in the historical transformation of English society and, corresponding with these, retain occupational norms related to their notions of professionalism. Even within Western societies there are reasons to believe that antecedent ideologies of professionalism rather than being completely replaced have simply been marginalized. Although clearly the modern occupational notion of professionalism is dominant now, there are sections of Western societies that continue to idealize professional norms of other types. It is this juxtaposition of elements from pre-modern, modern and postmodern ways of understanding professions, and the issues they deal with, that Lyon (1994) refers to as 'postmodernity'. Not only were modern and postmodern forms prefigured in the pre-modern (traditionalist), but the pre-modern has continued to be present, even if marginally, as society has changed. This mix has been highlighted by the global movement of social groups and the settlement by groups adhering to one world-view in societies where another is dominant.

The research conducted regarding the welfare perceptions of the Muslim community in Toronto offers compelling evidence of the vitality of occupational norms which would idealize non-modern forms of professionalism in welfare activity. Those sections of the Muslim community espousing an Islamic ideology of welfare maintained preferences regarding the characteristics of welfare agents which resemble in significant ways the outlook of religious professionalism described as dominant in medieval England. The medieval professional concerned with health and social care and the ideal welfare worker in the Muslim context are both sacred functionaries whose primary focus is on the 'cure of souls' and the preparation of souls for the afterworld. Both work within the purview of regulating sacred institutions. Sacred education and training are the primary requirements of both. Conversely, specialized knowledge and training are only secondary features, which are not deemed to be essential. Each perceives the welfare world in relationship to the community of belief. As a result, each is primarily focused on a specific community of belief and not upon humanity *per se*. As a corollary to this, any welfare activity offered beyond the boundaries of the community of belief is not understood as just welfare activity or even as primarily welfare activity but is clearly identified as missionary work.

Professional social work as peculiarly modern in character

The history of professionalism in England, reviewed above, would clearly indicate that modern social work is profoundly an expression of modern occupational professionalism (Parton, 1994). Indeed, what primarily distinguishes social work from other historical forms of welfare activity is that it has taken the idea of occupational professionalism and applied it to the welfare realm of human concern. By so doing it has been redefining the character of welfare activity according to the ideological outlook of the modern world-view. In this it has been so successful that, in the West at least, it has thoroughly marginalized previously dominant ideologies of welfare associated with earlier forms of professionalism and is attempting to do so now on the international stage. So much so, that social workers themselves have trouble recognizing any competing ideologies at all.

Reformulating the idea of professional imperialism

The review of competing welfare ideologies in the welfare situation of the Muslim community in Toronto, and the historical review of the parochially modern character of professionalism underlying contemporary social work, both would indicate that the social work profession is inescapably imperialistic in many situations of social diversity. Where social work embarks on serving populations which do not share its ideological outlooks on welfare it must be imperialistic, and no manner of superficial tinkering with social work's value base and professional activity can alter this. To cease to be imperialistic, social work would have to adopt alien ideologies of welfare fully, in which case it would necessarily cease to be a profession specializing in social relations, which amounts to no longer being what it uniquely and essentially is. Midgley's proposed solution of a pragmatic social work glosses over this reality.

Midgley's review of professional imperialism and his proposed solution feeds into a grand illusion to which professional social workers have been largely unconscious dupes for decades, the illusion being that professional social work is a universally valid expression of welfare activity which may legitimately transcend all barriers of diversity. Other ideologies of welfare, including the religiously-centred ones that were identified in the Islamic and the medieval English contexts, recognized ideological boundaries and were honest in recognizing that welfare activity beyond these were primarily missionary in character. Social work, under the illusion of secular universal validity, has not shown similar integrity. In a completely analogous situation social work has not recognized the missionary, or what I have been calling here the imperialistic, nature of its activity in situations of social diversity.

There are at least two compelling reasons for social workers to acknowledge the potentially missionary character of their profession. First and foremost, ethical consistency would seem to demand that a profession which claims to cherish the value of self-determination acknowledge realms of its activity which potentially impose upon this value. Second, where social workers are confronted by situations of social diversity it would seem critical for them to define their activities accurately, however unflattering that may be, for them to assess properly the impact of their interventions. Self-deception is not a virtue and is potentially very destructive in dealing with social realities.

The situation of ideological competition implicit in the Muslim minority community context in Toronto is again illustrative of the kind of consequences that this type of self-delusion can lead to for social work. One of the most striking findings emerging from the research conducted in to the welfare situation of the Muslim community in Toronto was the degree and tone of hostility that several respondents from the Muslim community indicated towards mainstream welfare services responding to wife abuse. Those respondents who were associated with the Islamic welfare ideology almost unanimously deemed all mainstream social services as missionary in character and hence counter-productive to the needs of Muslim women in abusive situations; because, along with offering logistic help, these services demanded, implicitly and sometimes explicitly, that these women abandon Islamic ideals they might retain. Emerging from this perception was the call for the development of Muslim community operated services which reflected some variation of Islamic welfare ideology.

For their part, it was clear that mainstream welfare respondents, including professional social workers, were not aware of the extent of the hostility maintained by these sections of the community, or were willing to dismiss their perceptions as illegitimate in the Canadian context. In this situation, mainstream welfare professionals could not, with utmost sincerity, conceive how their own activities could be perceived as an unwelcome intrusion by anyone who truly opposed wife abuse. The lack of awareness of these professionals contributed to the growth of inordinate hostility and sense of competition between welfare agents of the two communities and forestalled the possibility of any coordination of efforts.

Recognizing a missionary role

My argument in this paper has been that professional social workers have been unable to recognize perceptions of welfare phenomena other than their own because they simply have not acknowledged the possibility of multiple and competing ideologies of welfare persisting in situations of social diversity. Correspondingly, social workers have not acknowledged that their activities represent a form of missionary activity in many contexts of social diversity. Also, I have identified that this situation is ethically inconsistent for social work and counter-productive to the professed goals of social work activity. In response to the denial of the problem, and ongoing efforts to avoid it such as Midgley's call for a pragmatic social work, I propose that social work must make a conscious effort to acknowledge its missionary role and deal squarely with the consequences of this.

Practically speaking, to acknowledge the missionary character of social work is to recognize the presence of ideological boundaries for social work activity. When social work enters into situations of social diversity, it might be entering into the welfare space of another welfare ideology and may be setting itself up as a competitor to it. When social work advances into another ideology's space it should at the very least recognize that it is doing so, for it may severely impact on the kind of welfare relationships that it establishes both with individuals and with communities.

There are many minority communities in the West which chronically underutilize social work services, a problem which has usually been identified as one of 'access'. However, one explanation which cannot be ruled out is that many such communities simply do not accept the nature of social work services and therefore consciously and willingly try to avoid them. Traditional sections of the Muslim community in Toronto clearly represent an example of such communities. For these types of communities social work must simply accept the possibility that ideological boundaries with them are simply impermeable. Where the welfare ideology associated with social work is not welcome by a community no intrusion should be made into it, if at all avoidable. Similarly, on the international stage there are societies for which social work is simply inappropriate and for which no efforts should be made to advance social work activity.

There are, of course, many situations in the real world which compel social work activity over ideological boundaries. Such situations commonly arise in minority situations in the West, where weak minority communities have not been able to establish alternate welfare provision systems or are compelled by circumstances to employ state-sanctioned social work services. Also, in international situations social work is often introduced by Westernized ruling elites as part of modernization schemes. Traditional sectors of the society usually have very little say in these situations and are often compelled by force to accept the presence of international social work in their midst. In these situations social work must recognize that they are likely to be seen by traditional sectors of the community and society as missionaries for an alien ideology of welfare and a hostile world-view. Social work activity in these types of situations will be seen as a threat, which can lead to political tensions on many levels – within family, community and even society. In these types of situations social workers must learn to define the nature of their work bearing in mind ideological considerations. This would include the need to define the overall context of their practice in relation to community ideology and politics and to identify the kind of ideological barriers that may confront them. Also, with regard to individual clients that may emerge from such communities, social workers must be aware that relationships established or desired by the minority client likely will not correspond to the customary client–professional type of relationship. The social worker may be defining the relationship in accordance with customary patterns but the assumed client may in actuality be defining the relationship in accordance to patterns assumed from alternate welfare ideologies or in accordance to other practical considerations. Needless to say, knowing the actual nature of the relationship established or desired by assumed clients is essential if social workers are to assess properly the nature of their work in these situations and avoid self-delusion.

Summary and conclusions

The presence of diverging perceptions on the nature of welfare and welfare activity in the response to wife abuse in the Muslim community in Toronto revealed the phenomena of competing ideologies of welfare in situations of social diversity. The existence of competing welfare ideologies in this specific situation also uncovered the presence of competing perspectives on occupational norms and ideals for welfare provision, or what can be termed competing ideologies of professionalism. An historical review of the development of modern welfare professionalism revealed that the type of professionalism understood as normal and ideal by sections of the Muslim community in Toronto resembled in significant ways the type of professionalism found in earlier stages of the development of contemporary modern professionalism in the West.

The primary implication that was pursued and elaborated with regard to the social work profession was that modern notions of welfare and welfare professionalism are both parochial perspectives which can only be extended to communities manifesting competing perspectives at the cost of acknowledgeing a missionary or imperialistic stance to these communities. On the basis of this it was argued that the social work profession when operating in contexts of social diversity should acknowledge fundamental boundaries to the extension of its work in certain contexts of social diversity.

The identification of competing welfare ideologies in the situation of the Muslim community and the detailing of significant implications of these for the social work profession are indeed generalizable with regard to other social contexts and to the context of other health and social care professions.

It should be emphasized that the welfare situation of the Muslim minority community in Toronto is not an unusual one in the contemporary world. Social contexts where radically distinct communities confront one another in responding to welfare issues is increasingly common as communities of various types confront one another in today's increasingly complex and diverse world. Many communities for whom modern social welfare provision has been problematic likely retain ideological features which significantly impact upon their welfare relations with modern welfare institutions and professions. The severe problems that have faced the social work profession in its efforts to extend itself into the context of many traditional societies outside of the West can be related to some type of ideological competition (Azmi, 1994). Similarly, the many difficulties faced by social workers in the West in their efforts to provide effectively services to many minority communities may significantly relate to issues of ideological competition.

Also, the essentially modern character of professionalism in the context of social work similarly applies to all the contemporary health and social care professions. Specialization is the essential characteristic of modern epistemology. One of the consequences of specialization in the realm of occupational organization is occupational professionalism. A corresponding effect of specialization is the proliferation of narrowly focused professions which focus intensely on segregated realms of human activity. The secularization of the idea of welfare, and later its segregation into various realms, has related to the foundation of the various health and social professions. These various professional occupations cannot but represent activities which bring to effect the specific welfare ideology of the modern world-view, and parochially modern views of professionalism. Consequently, all health and social care professionals must realize that their activities represent the work of a specific ideological viewpoint, which in some cases may be radically at odds with the ideological viewpoint of diverse communities being served. Correspondingly, in situations of social diversity where alternate welfare ideologies are operational the activities of all health and social care professionals, such as those of social workers, inescapably maintain a missionary or imperialistic aspect.

The idea of secular and specialized types of care being administered through professional occupational forms is thought to give the contemporary health and social care occupations universal validity. The idea of a transcendent form of care is an alluring notion, but the evidence presented here would suggest that it represents a grand illusion. Care, like the idea of welfare it relates to, necessarily has ideological overtones which inescapably put it at odds with the competing formulations of similar phenomena from other ideological outlooks on welfare. In situations of social diversity health and social care professionals must be aware that they cannot separate their narrow concerns from wider ideological issues. The world of welfare interrelates and interconnects with wider phenomena in the rest of the world.

Like social workers, all health and social care professionals must acknowledge the potentially missionary character of their work in many situations of social diversity. To avoid self-delusion and potentially negative consequences they, like social workers, must come to grips with the idea that there exists fundamental boundaries to the portability of their professional work in many situations of social diversity.

References

Azmi, S. 1992: Traditional Islamic social welfare: its meaning, history, and contemporary relevance. In *Islamic Quarterly* **XXXV**, (3), 165–80; **XXXV**, (4), 209–24; **XXXVI**, (1), 28–45.

Azmi, S. 1994: Social welfare in the Muslim world: a case study of pre-revolutionary Iran. Paper presented at the Inter-University Consortium for International Social Development, 8th Biennial Symposium. Kandy, Sri Lanka.

Azmi, S. 1996: *Perceptions of the welfare response to wife abuse in the Muslim community of metropolitan Toronto.* Unpublished PhD thesis. Toronto: University of Toronto.

Blumer, H. 1966: Preface. In Vollmer, H.M. and Mills, D.L. (eds.) *Professionalization.* Englewood Cliffs, NJ: Prentice-Hall.

Elliott, P. 1972: *The sociology of the professions.* London: Macmillan.

Goldner, F.H., Ference, T.P. and Ritti, R.R. 1973: Priests and laity: a profession in transition. In Halmos, P. (ed.), *Professionalisation and social change.* Keele: University of Keele, 119–37.

Halmos, P. (ed.) 1973: *Professionalisation and social change.* Keele: University of Keele.

Hugman, R. 1991: *Power in caring professions.* London: Macmillan.

Kemp, C.F. 1947: *Physicians of the soul: a history of pastoral counselling.* New York: Macmillan.

Lubove, R. 1965: *The professional altruist: the emergence of social work as a career 1880–1930.* Cambridge, MA: Harvard University Press.

Lyon, D. 1994: *Postmodernity.* Buckingham: Open University Press.

McNeill, J.T. 1952: *A history of the cure of souls.* London: SCM Press.

Midgley, J. 1981: *Professional imperialism: social work in the Third World.* London: Heinemann.

Parton, N. 1994 'Problematics of government', (post)modernity and social work. *British Journal of Social Work* **24**(1), 9–32.

Rashdall, H. 1936: The medieval universities. In Powicke, F.M. and Emden, E.B. (eds), *The universities of Europe in the Middle Ages*, 3 volumes. Oxford: Clarendon Press.

Vollmer, H.M. and Mills, D.L. (eds.) 1966: *Professionalization.* Englewood Cliffs, NJ: Prentice-Hall.

Wilding, P. 1982: *Professional power and social welfare.* London: Routledge and Kegan Paul.

7

Social work and care in India

Gracy Fernandes and Kalindi Mazumdar

This chapter looks at concepts of care and their relationship to forms of professional social work in the multifaceted Indian cultural and economic contexts, with special reference to child and family welfare services.

The profession of social work in India has been largely derived from the US model in the first half of the twentieth century and had mostly a relief, remedial and rehabilitative approach. This was later understood to be inappropriate for the Indian sociocultural milieu with its pervasive poverty. Paradigm shifts were made, primarily in the late 1970s, in social work practice and education toward the promotion of economic development, the championing of human rights and the evolution of culturally appropriate approaches. Social work in India continues to develop along these lines.

The earliest formal professional training in social work in India dates back to 1936 (The Tata Institute of Social Sciences, Bombay) and was given by social work educators trained mostly in the United States and by a few who trained in Britain. These workers predominantly followed the psychosocial concepts of Western psychology and social dynamics. The rationale for this was the need to train social workers in the professional delivery of welfare and social services.

During the same period, several social reform movements were born in India, inspired by the ideals of their leaders, Mahatma Gandhi, Ambedkar, Mahatma Jyotiba Phule and E. Ramasami (affectionately called 'Periyar'), who attempted to achieve a level of social change for justice, and emancipation of women and the marginalized castes. It was believed that these changes in social attitudes would largely depend on the education of the people. Thus, untrained but highly motivated voluntary social workers began developmental work, such as literacy and awareness generation, income generation, and health education, using local resources. This work aimed to prevent social ills and disease and promote social change toward harmony, health, justice and economic well-being.

Unfortunately, although the social work profession was introduced to

India by people sympathetic with these social movements, the profession in India was neither incorporated by them nor did it incorporate them, and the profession remained stuck in an inappropriate Western model. Eventually, during the 1970s, the profession grasped the major shortcomings of the initial approach. The trained social workers dealt mainly with individual cases and thus performed a narrow role in society. Professional social work was unable to strike a resonant chord in the prevailing cultural milieu and promote social change (Bose, 1992; Ramachandran, 1988).

The shift toward a model for social change and development

The 1970s was a decade in which the worldwide attention that poverty and its social causes were receiving (*vide* Paulo Freire (1970) in Latin and South America, and Saul Alinsky (1972) in North America) did not escape the notice of Indian social work educators. They also recognized that in order for professional social work to have a significant impact on society it would have to involve itself in economic and social development:

> Our Curricula are derived from the residual remedial rehabilitative model of practice as they are largely borrowed from the West, mainly the U.S.A. Illustrative of this situation is that a majority of our curricula show emphasis on social and individual problems of pathology rather than problems of the individual and society in the context of *poverty and development*. Similarly, the curricula are *more urban than rural*, derived as they are, from a western, technologically oriented society. They are largely at the master's degree level when the need of the country is for large numbers of lower level workers (University Grants Commission, 1978, p. 298).

There was an urgency to redirect and integrate professional goals and academic content with the social realities of the country – poverty and injustice – and contribute to the social development of the people (Midgley, 1994). Relevant programmes at the Bachelor (undergraduate) and paraprofessional (high-school) levels were added.

In an earnest effort to redesign the social work curriculum and make it relevant to Indian social realities, the Curriculum Development Centre in Social Work Education chose to adopt the developmental approach while not neglecting the simultaneous need for remedial and rehabilitative services:

> The major task would be to promote *social change* and *development*, while recognising that groups or individuals already affected by the problems emanating from the structural factors in society will need help in meeting their immediate problems or needs. (University Grants Commission, 1990, p. 28).

Thus, traditional Western social work approaches were seen to be addressing curatively short-term needs and pathologies on a small scale, addressing individuals and families, while efforts directed at social change and development were viewed as necessary to address and prevent problems over the long term and on a larger scale in communities. There are now schools of social work in India that specialize in concentrating on social work methods related to field settings such as medical, child welfare, correctional, etc., while other schools offer a generic and integrated approach from the micro to the macro level.

Brigham (1982) recalls the story told to him by the British social work educator, Robin Huws-Jones. When he stopped at an Indian city to visit a young Indian woman alumna of his training program at Swansea, Wales, he had to stumble over dozens of recumbent people lying on the sidewalk outside the social worker's office. He was speechless when she proudly announced to him that she had managed to keep her monthly caseload to 35. Using this as an illustration, Brigham further comments:

> In India, with perhaps the most sizeable, complex and pervasive social problems in the world, the notion that one-to-one or even one-to-a-family work can provide amelioration, let alone solutions, is patently ludicrous. Clearly, as social work educators in India are now stating, there needs to be a focus on social change; on *social* development; on the systems approach; on work with villages, tribes, organisations, communities and co-operatives; on programs for families, youth, children, women and the aged (p. 71).

Like Jamshidi (1978), Brigham suggests that casework and the clinical approach need to be placed in proper perspective as part of the function social workers are taught to perform.

To heighten the impact of social work, professional associations were soon formed, such as the Indian Association of Social Workers and the various state-level and metropolitan associations of social workers, which were able to give a vocal backing to the individual advocacy and lobbying efforts of social workers, on behalf of the masses, for social change and development. Lobbying and advocacy were found to be a necessary part of professional social work in India. Despite the legally framed policy intentions of the government to uplift the disadvantaged and promote development (especially in the areas of child and family welfare, in health, nutrition, education and income generation) social workers and others have long-cited the lack of political will on the part of government at the various levels to bring about decisively the necessary changes for a just society. On account of this lack, development, particularly of the marginalized social groups, has been delayed (Weiner, 1991).

Networking forums where various other helping professions could share concerns and insights emerged, such as the Women's Forum, Campaign Against Child Labour, Forum Against Child Sexual Exploitation, Forum for Social Advocacy and several people's movements for community development. International legal documents such as the Convention on the Rights of the Child and statistics on social indicators of development published by the United Nations Development Programme (UNDP), United Nations Educational Scientific and Cultural Organization (UNESCO) and International Labour Organisation (ILO) are strong and persuasive tools used by the voluntary sectors to mobilize the government to enact and enforce legislation and implement programmes in favour of the vulnerable sections of society.

As a result of the above activities professional social work is better recognized in society and by the government. Professionally trained social workers today are employed by the Indian government as probation officers in juvenile homes, as community development officers in the municipalities, as medical social workers in family planning centres and as counsellors, motivators and social workers in municipal schools and in social welfare programmes for backward classes in rural areas. Remaining problems are bureaucratization and lack of accountability and conviction in the possibility of social change in government agencies, a lack which tends to stymie creativity and zeal and thus tends to reduce the quality of work (Weiner, 1991).

The growing awareness in government of the need for more agencies, especially to reach disadvantaged women and children, prompted it to invite the voluntary sector to collaborate with it by subcontracting welfare programmes to non-governmental organizations (NGOs), offering technical, managerial and partial financial support to these organizations. This initiative generated a rapid growth of new NGOs from the 1970s onwards, working in rural development, social activism and social advocacy. Many of the NGOs were founded by social workers, sometimes beginning under the wing of schools of social work as innovative field demonstration programmes.

The ongoing challenges to the social work profession today include increasing poverty, inadequate government social expenditure, lack of access to education and health care, problems due to the inequality of women in society, the lingering caste system and urban–rural disparities. All these occur within a multifaceted and rapidly changing cultural, social, economic and political scenario (Thurz and Vigliante, 1975).

Reinterpretation of social work concepts in the Indian milieu

To achieve the desired social changes, social workers have become increasingly aware of the need for socio-culturally, economically and politically appropriate methods and have been developing new concepts of care. Already there is a growing wealth of knowledge, practice wisdom and competence in the hundreds of projects and people's movements across the country, demonstrating innovative entrepreneurship, but these are not yet well-documented.

In the rest of this chapter we will discuss cultural appropriateness in social work practice in India and then we will examine approaches to community development, with a special focus on children and women.

Working in a culturally appropriate manner

India is a land of diverse religions, languages, castes, cultures and wide economic disparities. For social work practice to be meaningful in the Indian context, it is imperative that it identify and consider the importance of cultural factors operating in the life of the multi-ethnic Indian society. Mukundarao (1969) perceives these at two levels: at the first level culture is normative and inspirational because it is based on the ancient legacy of thought and vision; and at the second level it governs 'the common codes and modes of behaviour'. Social work can draw on the first level to motivate clients, while at the second level professional practice is tested in the actual and existential life situation.

Universal human experiences, such as birth, certain developmental milestones, social behaviours and the sharing of joy and sorrows, are similar across various cultures. There are, however, other factors which are unique to each culture, such as family dynamics, social structures, communications styles, religious beliefs and rituals. Manoleas (1994) describes this fact as 'human sameness versus difference'.

Several Indian social work educators (trained in the United States and later teaching and practising in India) have realized the significance of the cultural variants in social work practice. They have emphasized the need to build up a body of indigenous literature on appropriate social work practice, incorporating Indian thought and reflecting Indian philosophy, tradition of work and perception of needs, in order to indigenize social work practice and education (Banerjee, 1972; Mathew, 1992; Mukundarao, 1969; Nagpaul, 1967; Thangavelu, 1978; University Grants Commission, 1978).

There is a need for the social worker to be able to think and reflect on the cultural situation before determining the best course of action to help clients, instead of mechanically and routinely applying techniques taken from the West. It is useful for the social worker to document experiences methodically: portraying clearly, concisely and vividly the client's situation and explaining the rationale for a course of action. Documentation and sharing of experiences among social workers helps build up the knowledge, skill and value base for appropriate social work.

The major cultural factors to be considered in the Indian context are related primarily to the following:

- the concepts of autonomy, self-determination, the questioning of authority, confidentiality and other social work principles;
- the client–worker relationship;

- the individual, the family and the community;
- the role of informal care;
- the use of cultural beliefs, symbols, traditions and communication media to change attitudes;
- health interventions by the social worker.

The concepts of autonomy, self-determination, the questioning of authority, confidentiality and other social work principles

Social work educators and practitioners tend to take for granted such goal-concepts of social work as individual autonomy, self-determination, direct expression of emotions, assertiveness, objectivity and the questioning of authority. Similarly taken for granted is the maintenance of confidentiality by the social worker of the client's problems. Students of social work especially take these goals to their field practice and analyse their 'cases' against these 'accepted' principles. Students are less flexible than are seasoned workers and often they apply principles literally.

These goals suggest a particular Western psychosocial, political perspective in which value is placed on the individual competing freely within existing legal, economic and social institutions. This runs counter to Indian realities and cultural beliefs, which emphasize respect for tradition and deference to authority, family cooperation over individual achievement, community interdependence and the diverse religious philosophies and traditions prevailing in the country (Rhodes, 1991) .

In India, for the most part, social work professionals belong to the upper and middle economic classes, are often fairly Westernized and to an extent are out of touch with the culture of the communities they work in. So, to be effective, social work practitioners need to be aware of the culture in which they are working, of the culture from whence social work concepts are derived, and at the same time be aware of their own socio-cultural 'baggage' or background. The prerequisite for the client and social worker pair for working through difficult life situations, whether in meeting immediate survival needs or in achieving emotional well-being, is the knowledge of self, both of the social worker and of the client (Banerjee, 1972). The cultural dimension of social work is increasingly discussed now, but there is little literature on this dimension (Banerjee, 1972; Manoleas, 1994; Mathew, 1992; Mukundarao, 1969; Nagpaul, 1972).

Child rearing in Western and Indian societies is a good example of the differences in the two cultural systems. Erikson's psychosocial stages of child development indicate how the socio-cultural environment marks the formative characteristics such as the parent–child relationship of dependency compared with independence, or assertiveness compared with submission. In addition, a large family discourages individuality and breeds in the child a feeling of being just one of the group. This works against the achievement of a 'self' distinct from others (Sinha, 1981). All this is especially evident in the case of the Indian girl child, who grows up knowing her 'place' with respect to males.

The role and status of women is an equally important area of cultural difference to note because women form the majority of the client-group approaching social work agencies for child and family welfare services and they play an important role in caring as the main caregivers in the family. Indian society is largely male-dominated and patriarchal: authoritarian attitudes in daily life can lead to the oppression of women and children. For example, the Indian woman who dare not utter her husband's name at the time of intake will equate the concepts of equality and autonomy with disrespect to her husband because she is subordinated to the male authority of her husband.

Group formation of poor women is a means of empowering women to change the situation of male domination, because here they can begin to open up and discuss their problems in a supportive environment. This is useful, for example, in projects that give poor women earning opportunities because often men become hostile to the women's attempts to control their income; the men may work less and yet be unwilling to take on some of the household work (Krishnaraj, 1996).

The client–worker relationship

The US model teaches that the heart of casework is the client–worker relationship (Perlman, 1957). Also, in India, a rapport of trust is essential in casework. In the Indian context this is built through the communication of a caring attitude over a period of time. Additionally, for an effective outcome, the social worker tries to help the client develop his or her self-worth, dignity and potential so that the 'dependency syndrome' does not persist.

Professional social workers in India, like the early Friendly Visitors of the nineteenth century in the United States, assume that those who enter their profession do so out of altruistic motives. They also assume that with their professional knowledge and expertise they can 'do good' to their clients. Later on they developed the theory of the helping process and planned interventions to empower their clients.

Today in India there are still many child and family welfare programmes based on the idea of benevolence and focus on 'doing good' for others in need, for example, some of the programmes of international child sponsorship. In this type of set-up, the client–worker relationship is one of receiver–giver. There is a need to change this type of client–worker relationship because it causes dependency, not development. However, the basic current philosophy of child sponsorship is to enable the family and later the child to become self-sufficient and it is precisely this which tests the social worker's skills in moving the adult members of the family creatively towards economic independence as proved in the lives of numbers of families.

On the other hand, the pervasive perception the poor, uneducated clients have of the social worker is that of someone with the power to 'do good' – an authoritative, knowledgeable, expert, a giver of resources. In India, poor people often speak of an educated person, including social workers and politicians, as being like a 'mother' or a 'father' to them. This perception engenders the fear of asking questions, of suggesting other ways of doing things. This is an obstacle to participation and reinforces the top-down planning approach.

To counter this perception, the social worker must employ much effort and skill to motivate clients to think and act for themselves and participate in the helping process. The social worker can thus become a catalyst for change instead of a 'do-gooder'. One problem encountered by social work educators in trying to emphasize the concept of the social worker as catalyst is that many of the students who enter this field are less thinkers and persuaders and more doers, women and men of action, which is in large part a product of the Indian educational system. Social work educators need patiently to try to change this orientation of the students.

The heart of social problems in India is the powerlessness of the people, especially the lower caste groups. A directive and formal approach is not appropriate as it will tend only to further alienate clients who perceive social workers as authority figures and who address them as *Shetji* or *Memsaheb* (Sir or Madam). To gain the trust and confidence of the people social workers must demonstrate a respect for people's inherent human worth and dignity. Use of a non-directive, non-formal approach helps to achieve this. To illustrate: the use of appropriate language, seating arrangements – either all on the floor or all on chairs, not just the worker sitting on the chair and the client on the floor – or accepting a cup of tea offered as a sign of hospitality on a home visit are important gestures of conveying respect, acceptance and equality, qualities which characterize caring.

The social worker also needs to demonstrate a non-judgmental attitude with clients. Awareness of one's own values helps in the maintenance of a non-judgmental attitude to the values of others. Ideas of punctuality, personal cleanliness and propriety have a meaning to the middle-class professional, yet often poor clients will come to see the social worker at their convenience, without respecting the appointed time; lack of water supply and poverty affect the ability of a person to be 'presentable'. The social worker must avoid expressions of surprise or revulsion, as these may lead to lack of trust in the caring attitude of the worker. In the area of health care, values surrounding family planning and abortion are delicate and easily become religious conflicts in Muslim and Christian communities.

Owing to resource constraints, social workers may not be able to address the numerous needs of the clients; however, just being with them expresses caring, and clients can sense this.

The individual, the family and the community

The individual is strongly bound to family ties and is influenced by parental, or husband's, authority even in routine details. The client is more influenced by the family and social group than by the caseworker, at least initially, and thus the caseworker has to know the situation and how to deal with it by being 'an observer, a manipulator and a participant in relationships' (Banerjee, 1972). A woman, for example, will not easily make commitments to the worker without first obtaining her husband's consent, especially in the lower economic strata of society. The family approach is often more appropriate than the individual approach. The strengths of the family need to be viewed as assets in supporting and providing the individual with resources to meet situational stress and problems.

The family as a unit of social organization is an important value for the individual. It should be remembered that 'family' often means 'extended family', whether living together or not. The social worker should be aware of what various relational terms mean in a particular context: for example, 'brother' or 'sister' can include cousins. Today, joint families of over 200 members are rare, and usually consist of three generations living under the same roof, possibly including the families of two or three brothers. Families, however, are becoming increasingly nuclearized.

With the breakdown of the traditional systems of social support, such as the joint family, especially with urbanization, there has been a growing awareness that professional organizations and institutions need to play a greater role in caring for the handicapped, the aged, the homeless and the destitute. For example, in view of the millions of children who leave their impoverished and sometimes broken homes in rural areas for the streets of cities where they hope to find employment, social workers in NGOs today are offering them shelter, literacy, health education and job training in non-institutional settings.

In tribal cultures in India there is still a strong pattern of interdependence and reciprocity among individuals, families and the tribes. There is a growing body of knowledge accumulated by Indian anthropologists, notably on the tribal population, culture and economy, which is emphasized in the present day to promote and protect the human rights of tribal communities.

Everywhere in India, but particularly in cities, characterized by large, highly heterogeneous populations, social workers have to be sensitive to and respectful of this diversity. With the upsurge of religious fundamentalism in India, with its wake of riots and killings, social workers try to develop mutual respect and communal harmony between the different groups through creative street-plays and consultation in neighbourhood peace committees. Teachers and social workers in schools are being trained by social work educators to create awareness in children and college students about communal issues through classroom discussions.

Holistic approaches

In view of the above, whole-community and whole-person approaches are more relevant than those that view the client from a narrow perspective. The problems encountered by individuals, families and communities in India are largely generated by structural problems in the national economic and social system, such as unemployment or unstable employment with low wages, inadequate and deteriorating housing and lack of access to health care. These problems are intertwined and interconnected and logically suggest integrated solutions. Case management will, then, form the major component of the current mainstream of social work practice in India.

Additionally, when the whole person is considered in his or her full social context, he or she is seen not as an anonymous client, only a recipient of services, but as a person who may well have something to give. Reciprocity is an essential part of the structure and functioning of effective services and of empowerment.

Social workers must be able to plan a broad spectrum of services which are flexible, coherent and easy to use in reaching and helping the most disadvantaged children and families. They will also be able to cross traditional professional expectations and bureaucratic boundaries if the needs of those served are at stake. Programme planning and service delivery will see the child in the context of the family and the family in the context of its surroundings and provide continuity and communicate a sense of respect and caring (Schorr, 1989).

The skills of the social worker as an enabler and facilitator will include case finding, assessment, goal setting, care planning, networking, service implementation, monitoring and evaluation.

Below we give a brief description of a model of casework (the Samsar model) adapted to the Indian situation developed two decades ago. We include this model to make the reader aware of the types of cultural factors that the Indian social worker may have to take into consideration. The profession of social work in India, however, is not widely familiar with this model.

Today the Samsar model would no longer be relevant to those more urbanized and Westernized areas where Indian traditions are weaker. A shift in values corresponding to the breakdown of the extended family, toward individualism, has also been noted, and is reflected in Indian cinema. Even in the slums, many clients would rather be helped to identify the alternative choices before them than to accept advice. They may not believe in God or be swayed by traditional cultural beliefs or they may not even uphold the value of harmony in the family over their own individual desires, as this model tries to do. A typical case today, as 20 years ago, is that of a young woman desiring to marry or eloping outside her caste and finding resistance from her family. The family is likely to be the agent to contact the social worker. Today the girl is more likely to go ahead with the marriage.

Sometimes the social worker has to help the couple to avoid joint suicide in the face of family opposition to the marriage.

The Samsar model of casework
The Samsar model of casework is based on an holistic understanding of Indian life, psychology and culture – the classical Indian philosophy of the Hindu–Buddhist tradition, the caste system, class, regional differences, family structure, arranged marriages, the dowry system, religious beliefs, the theories of karma (fate, reward) and dharma (duty, harmony), various superstitions, astrology, horoscopes, palmistry and other such factors. Thangavelu (1978), who worked with the noted anthropologist Margaret Mead, has also formulated a syllabus to teach the Samsar model. This model, however, does not challenge social customs as much as it strives to seek the harmonious adjustment of the individual to the prevailing social situation. It works in harmony with whatever informal care the family avails of, such as the advice of a local religious leader or an astrologer.

Samsar means family. In contrast to the classical Western casework model, the unit of attention in India is not the client but the client's family. This is appropriate because major decisions in the family are usually taken by the eldest male and additionally there are specific roles prescribed for each of the other family members, especially in extended families, for example, for the eldest son, the eldest daughter, the mother-in-law, the daughter-in-law and so on. This model has an ecological perspective of society, which views the physical and social environments as shaping and being shaped by culture.

The casework process in the Samsar model   The helping process is divided into four stages: preparation, choice of points of entry, intervention and termination of the contract.

At the preparation stage the worker first assesses the situation and the consequences of transactions. She or he studies the covert and the overt factors. She or he meets the family members involved in the situation and reaches an agreement on the priorities in the problem and makes a verbal contract.

At the choice of points of entry, the social worker then intervenes at different levels, that is, by helping the individual member or the family members or both. This intervention is based on Indian cultural factors, for instance, respect for elders.

Active intervention is the next step whereby specific tasks are performed by the client and the worker. The worker helps the client in the performance and fulfilment of these tasks. A direct, advice-giving approach is encouraged, where the client is open to such an approach.

In the process of intervention, the worker is direct and uses her or his knowledge of Indian life to offer help in tune with the client's social milieu. The goal is to produce a growth-inducing fit between the client and his or her environment.

The social worker is exhorted continually to put into practice Indian philosophical concepts in order to improve her or his functioning. Certain concepts from Indian philosophy are used to help counsel clients, for example, the stages of life defined in the Indian scriptures, the theories of karma and dharma, the concept of Naya (the illusion of this life) and the cyclical concepts of time and space. Accordingly, nothing is everlasting and all events are cyclical. Thus a client who is suffering physically and mentally can be helped to realize the cyclical concept of life, for example, that his or her misery will pass away; as happiness and misery are cyclical.

It is culturally understood that the worker will not take sides. In marital problems, even though individual interviews are conducted with each spouse, the worker helps them as a couple to preserve family life.

The last step is the termination of the contract and an evaluation of the client's functioning. Thangavelu states that, in the final analysis, life cannot be framed into a system or be compartmentalized. Knowledge offered equips the client to meet life in all its variety and depth.

The role of informal care

Traditional forms of informal care in the family and the community (informal care, charity) have not challenged the rigid social structure of the caste system and thus have been unable to root out age-old social inequalities and injustices, yet traditional forms of informal care remain important because of their credibility with the community. Although social work educators recognize the need for formal training they also emphasize the need to recognize the important role played by informal care and the need to work with it.

Informal care has been strong in the disadvantaged caste communities and this demands that social work practitioners be very sensitive to the strengths and weaknesses of informal care in any given situation.

The recognition of informal care is of prime importance and has considerable implications for the way in which formal social work practice and services and the role of the trained social workers are viewed.

It is necessary to consider how best the formal services can be organized to fit in with and support informal care. From this perspective social work agencies cannot be conceived as sophisticated centres of service delivery given by social service providers to the poor and needy; rather, one asks how best social work agencies can be integrated into the culturally specific realities of the population in the process of social development.

There is a need for knowledge of different cultural caregiving patterns within families, kinship networks and communities in caring for the young, the infirm, the aged, the mentally ill and the physically and mentally handicapped. An holistic approach of 'the person in his or her environment' focuses on cultural norms of informal caring by families and communities.

Knowledge of tribal culture and social network analysis is essential in assessing resources and supports for family members, particularly women, prior to formulating problem statements or intervention plans, because of strong tribal bonds and the accepted belief in witchcraft.

In locally-based work there needs to be a profound respect for the integrity of the local culture. Often the grass-roots-level workers belong to the area and are known by the community and in turn they know the community. There is value and validity of such workers doing 'ordinary tasks' and acting as intermediaries and bridges between professional formal care and informal care. A vital aspect of the services is being accessible to vulnerable people who may shy away from a large-scale, impersonal and formal type of care. To achieve this, workers who are more like the beneficiaries of the services are likely to be more effective than people who are unlike the beneficiaries (Repetto, 1977).

The use of cultural beliefs, symbols, traditions and communications media to change attitudes

Advanced psychoanalytical theory has been used by Kakar (1978, 1979) to interpret motifs of Indian myths and legends to give social workers a better understanding of how basic Indian culture may affect client perceptions. Social work educators such as Banerjee, Mukundarao and Nagpaul have emphasized that insights into the deep-rooted beliefs, symbols and traditions of Indian culture can be applied to achieve social change to counter passive acceptance and fatalism.

There will be situations in which the social worker can appeal to the client's sense of dharma (duty), to persuade him or her to give up problem behaviours, or in which the worker can rationally convey the facts about how a problem can be remedied and help the client to overcome despair and fatalism. The majority of the Indian population will be receptive to this type of approach to their problems (Mathew, 1992).

Knowledge of how culture affects basic developmental events such as gender roles, rites of passage, sexuality development, mate selection, child-rearing practices, social networks, ageing and mourning helps in planning interventions.

For the future survival and development of rural and tribal populations, their traditional protective role toward nature needs to be strengthened in the face of the depletion of forest resources as a result of population pressure and the greed of urban-based timber trade and industrial development.

The use of various folk media to communicate with and involve client communities, such as street-plays, folk theatre, storytelling, puppetry, dance drama and songs can help to communicate concepts and ideas to clients. Musical clips from Indian films are a popular source of attraction and are used creatively as a tool to initiate discussion on social issues such as marriage, the status of women, inequalities in society and other issues. Illiteracy need not be a barrier to communication if popular oral methods enlivened by visual aids are used. The various communication strategies are informative, instructive as well as entertaining and have been effective in literacy campaigns and particularly in educating groups of children, youth, women and communities about the relatively complex health issues of HIV and AIDS.

Health interventions by the social worker

Given the shortage of trained medical personnel, social workers in India, especially in the villages, need to be able to assess health, illness, functional and dysfunctional behaviour and psychopathology, taking into account the cultural relativity of categories and modes of expression. These same concepts are useful for medical personnel as well, when available. Religious networks and local-based networks are sources of aid in many rural communities, where formal health services are unavailable, unreliable or inadequate.

Social workers in medical and psychiatric settings assess the clients from an holistic perspective and take into account the folk concepts of mental illness and its management. For example, treatment for mental illness according to folk beliefs may consist of a combination of several treatments administered together, such as spiritual and occult rituals, medicines, special diet, exercises and massage (Balodhi, 1991). Other treatment may include physical violence to the mentally ill patient to exorcize the evil spirits. Clients need to be defended against harmful practices, but those that are not harmful need not be discouraged by the social worker.

When working in urban slums or rural areas, social workers with a middle-class health consciousness must be aware of the locally held traditional beliefs and practices surrounding illnesses, such as measles, chicken pox and polio, which are interpreted by these people as 'visitations of the Goddess' and hence not to be treated medically. The fact that this may result in the child's death or disability, indicates the need for the social worker to change the thinking of the people.

Knowledge of and sensitivity to traditional health and spiritual practices that have been proven beneficial through restoring harmony in the individual can help the social worker to plan appropriate interventions. Some of the physical exercise techniques such as Yoga and Vipassana (a Buddhist self-awareness technique that helps achieve a happy useful life) have been introduced in prison settings (for example, in the Tihar Jail, New Delhi, by the noted police officer and Mangsaysay Award winner, Ms Kiran Bedi).

The neglect of the health of girls compared with that of boys is another area of concern for the social worker who has to counter the culturally conditioned preferred treatment given to male children in terms of diet and health care. The importance of health and nutritional awareness and care for women and especially antenatal care are also areas where the social worker needs to place emphasis, since in India, women are reluctant to discuss or seek care for their gynaecological health problems and they tend to believe that pregnancy and childbirth are natural events that do not need medical care, yet maternal and infant mortality remain fairly high (Arasu, 1990; Mahadevan, 1985; UNICEF, 1990).

The child-to-child approach to health education is based on the fact that older children are made to care for their younger children at home while their mothers work. Attractive health fairs are arranged for the children where they learn through puppet shows, songs and dances. Children's groups are formed for more in-depth learning. Later on, mothers' workshops are organized where the children teach the mothers, because the link to the mother in health-awareness generation is useful.

Working in socio-economic and political dimensions: towards development

In a country with such widespread poverty as India, a community view or approach is necessary for effective social change. Schools of social work exhort social workers to take on a developmental, preventive role, empowering people for self-help in meeting basic needs and reorientating the values of the community – raising the value of the girl child and the woman, promoting the development of the child and encouraging cooperation among the castes. Priority areas for services include the poorest, most disadvantaged, remote and isolated communities.

Within the community approach there is a place for the use of all the traditional social work methods of individual casework, group work and community organization and social activism. As always, the client–worker relationship is central to gaining the confidence and the trust of the community. If the goal of social work is the promotion of a quality of life, then social workers need to possess skills and techniques to enable families and communities to achieve the desired development. The skills required stretch from individual interviewing and therapy skills to interpersonal communication skills for social advocacy and lobbying. Skills in planning, administration, research and social welfare policy analysis are useful for workers who are promoted upwards from direct-service positions (Gilbert and Specht, 1986).

New skill and knowledge areas being introduced in schools of social work include legal literacy, knowledge of international and national instruments of human rights, social planning, economics, structural analysis, political systems and management skills such as conflict resolution and disaster management.

Social activists in India are increasingly focusing on helping people realize the source of their alienation in the larger society and organize them to take action. This has a political dimension. It is now understood that palliative solutions are no longer the answer.

A typical social work setting is that of the urban slum, where social workers are involved in poverty upliftment programmes. Schemes of city governments and builders which offer to compensate slum dwellers for their homes in exchange for leaving the area often see slum dwellers ending up with more money than they have ever seen, but homeless, and soon the money is frittered away. Social workers empower slum dwellers to make the right decision by warning them of this likely consequence and advising them to improve their living conditions where they are. The residents face the dilemma of choosing to believe the caring professional social workers or accepting the deceptively attractive offer of the builders, while social workers maintain a non-directive approach.

This and some other situations demonstrate that the problems lie deeper than the traditional skills and resources of the social worker. The venturing of the profession into conflict situations, such as forest conservation versus rights of the forest dwellers, developmental industrial projects versus the right of farmers to land, bring to light the contradictory patterns of care and development paradigms.

Glimpses of professional social work in such situations are also seen in major social movements and their constructs, for example, in the Narmada Bachao Andolan (Save the Narmada Movement), the Chipko (Hug the Trees) Movement (Bahuguna, 1994) and the Harit Vasai (Green Vasai) Movement. Most of these movements began with the inspiration of untrained, concerned, committed citizens who later realized the need for using trained social workers. Some of these workers came on student placement and were later employed. An essential feature of these movements is the people's participation in analysing current issues affecting the community and in designing strategies. Another movement is Samarathan, working with tribal and other rural populations. These movements are slowly evolving to embrace the current socio-political scenarios of an ever turbulent Indian society.

Hallmarks of today's movements and development efforts include mobilising women and youth against alcoholism and illicit distilleries, to form cooperatives and obtain government loan savings and credit schemes and technical assistance and to work together to build rural infrastructure. A well-known example is the work of Anna Hazare, in whose 'ideal village' model villagers come to accept prohibition, family planning, community farming through *shramdan* (voluntary labour), cattle grazing and afforestation programmes (Kokje, 1996; Murthy,1989; Times of India News Service, 1996). Some NGOs specialize in training, especially using the participatory approach in action, research and advocacy. These also emphasize the importance of the roles of women and children in participation in health, education, economic and social development, the underlying philosophy being summed up in the maxim: people cannot be developed by others, they can only develop themselves (Sridharan, 1993; Younghusband, 1968). In this light several international child-sponsorship agencies have been trying out community development approaches since the 1970s. Community-based organizers are made responsible for securing basic necessities for the community such as water, sanitation and garbage disposal and for organizing literacy drives, nursery schools, and so on. Efforts to improve employment and self-employment for parents are also made by the social workers of these agencies (Fernandes *et al.*, 1995).

At the same time there are several special interest and political groups and parties vying for the allegiance of the people for political and/or economic gains. In view of this, in order to keep alive the noble ideals of caring, the social work profession needs the enduring commitment of educators, administrators, practitioners and students to continue asking, 'For whom?' and 'How?' when planning interventions, social advocacy and policy.

The life and work of the social reformers of the first half of the twentieth century Mahatma Gandhi, Ambedkar, Mahatma Jyotiba Phule and E. Ramasami 'Periyar', continue to be important sources of inspiration to participants in today's social movements, as lower caste and indigenous populations (tribal and others) have been inspired by them and are becoming more vocal and visible on the political scene (Fernandes, 1984; Nahar and Chandani, 1995).

In view of this, it is worth recalling some of the features of the Indian Sarvodaya Movement, which is an holistic Indian model of village development or 'constructive work', theorized by Mahatma Gandhi, Vinobha Bhave, Jay Prakash Narayan and others. Sarvodaya, meaning the welfare and enlightenment of all, was based on morality, non-violence and concepts of justice. It aimed at the holistic development of villages to make them self-sufficient, since they form the basis of Indian economy and social life. The uplifting of women was an important focus of the Sarvodaya movement, which saw them organized into groups, beginning to earn and participating in the governance of the village. The education of children was to be practical as well as academic to prepare them for a creative role in the future of the village.

Sarvodaya envisioned a voluntary social worker entering a village, sharing the life of the people and functioning as a *teacher* through personal example as well as through formal and informal teaching. The areas of emphasis were on hygiene and sanitation to prevent disease, the protection and development of the natural environment, the development of handicrafts, the development of the human personality through practical, academic, physical and spiritual education, the elimination of untouchability and changes in unjust economic relationships (Gandhi, 1958; Mashruwala, 1958).

Obstacles such as the pervasiveness of the caste system, especially the system of untouchability, and some economic and political factors have hampered the movement from spreading widely. There is the grim fact that many villages have fallen into the grip of political parties (as vote banks) and that adherence to one religion or the other has become an excuse for division among the people in many urban and rural areas.

Yet, in today's India the influence of Sarvodaya is seen in the conceptual basis of rural development education in institutes of management, schools of social work, government programmes and a number of new movements and NGOs in India. (Muttagi, 1986; Nair and Ambarasan, 1981; Reddy, 1991; Shepard, 1987). Additionally, it inspired a vibrant movement in Sri Lanka that currently engages the energies of people in a few thousand villages. The principles of Buddhism and methodical decentralization were introduced in the Sri Lankan movement by A.T. Ariyaratna who had earlier participated in the Indian Sarvodaya movement (Macy, 1985).

Development efforts both by government and by NGOs consciously focus on planning and designing programmes for women and children at individual, community and macro levels. The task forces who drew up the national plans of action of the Indian government for children and women included faculties of schools of social work and other professionals. The plan of action for the child sought to promote the basic survival and the development of the child. The areas of priority emphasized were prenatal and postnatal care, health, nutrition, immunization, availability of potable water, primary education and a secure family environment for the child. The plan for women specified reproductive health care, non-formal education, income generation, women's-group organization, basic legal and political literacy, and representation in the local governments (DWCD, 1992). Protection of the rights of women and children was also a stated goal. Various human rights organizations are lobbying to enforce international human rights instruments and labour laws protecting women and children, their dignity and worth.

Conclusions

This chapter has examined concepts of care in social work practice in India and considered the suitability of the Western model of social work to the constantly metamorphosing Indian social realities. It has explored areas for developing culturally, socially, economically and politically adequate theoretical frameworks and concepts related to the rich Indian heritage.

Social work educators recognize the need to present students with wisdom distilled from an in-depth effort of reflection on experiences in social work practice, not merely with simplified parallel applications between the Western and Eastern situations. The values, knowledge and skills thus imparted will truly be appropriate to the Indian context.

Today's challenges demand a response from the social work profession to engage more actively in participatory development and to focus attention more effectively on the poorest and most disadvantaged groups in society, particularly women and children, through both service and advocacy.

Working in the spirit of dharma (duty), today's Indian social workers can be inspired by the teachings of Swami Vivekananda of Calcutta (1802–1902), the well-known religious and social reformer, who emphasized that the *opportunity to help is to be valued more than the possibility of reward*, a concept in line with the Baghavad Gita (Patel, 1987). He rejected the lingering age-old casteist view of the poor and disadvantaged that tended to underlie social injustices. Observing the distortion of values in the callousness of his society, he attempted to galvanize the youth into action with the words

> So long as the millions live in hunger and ignorance, I hold every man a traitor who, having been educated at their expense, pays not the least heed to them.

References

Alinsky, S.D. 1972: *Rules for radicals*. New York: Vintage Books.

Arasu, K. 1990: Gender based malnutrition and mortality in India. *Grassroots Action* 3 (special issue on the girl child); 49–52.

Banerjee, G.R. 1972: *Papers on social work, an Indian perspective*. Series 23. Bombay: Tata Institute of Social Sciences.

Bahuguna, S.L. 1994: *Whither development?* Silgara, Tihri Garhwal: Chipko Information Centre, Parvatiya Navjivan Mandal.

Balodhi, J.P. 1991: Holistic approach to psychiatry: the Indian view. *National Institute of Mental Health and Neurosciences Journal* 9(2), 101–4.

Bose, A.B. 1992: Social work in India: developmental roles for a helping profession. In Hohenstad, M.C., Khinduka, S.K and, Midgley, J. (eds), *Profiles in international social work*. Washington: National Association of Social Workers Press.

Brigham, T. 1982: Social work in five developing countries: relevance of US microsystems model. *Journal of Education for Social Work* 18(2),

DWCD 1992: *National plan of action – a commitment to the child*. New Delhi: Department of Women and Child Development.

Fernandes, W. 1984: *Social activists and people's movements*. New Delhi: Indian Social Institute.

Fernandes, G., Bakshi, A. and Mehta, N. 1995: *An evaluation of the impact of sponsorship-aid provided by CASP-PLAN in the resettlement area of Malad East (Bombay)*. Bombay: Research Unit, College of Social Work.

Freire, P. 1970: *Pedagogy of the oppressed*. Harmondsworth: Penguin Books.

Gandhi, M.K. 1958: A model zamindar; village work. In Kumarappa, B. (ed.), *Sarvodaya: the welfare of all*. Ahmedabad: Navajivan Publishing House.

Gilbert, N. and Specht, H. 1986: *Dimensions of social welfare policy*. Englewood Cliffs, NJ: Prentice-Hall.

Jamshidi, L. 1978: Casework in developing nations. *Journal of Education for Social Work* 14(2), 46–52.

Kakar, S. 1978: *The inner world: a psycho-analytic study of childhood and society in India*. New Delhi: Oxford University Press.

Kakar, S. 1979: *Indian childhood: cultural ideals and social reality*. New Delhi: Oxford University Press.

Kokje, M. 1996: They no more venture out to greener pastures. *Times of India* 16 March.

Krishnaraj, M. 1996: Women's empowerment alone is not enough. *Times of India* 6 March.

Macy, J. 1985: Dharma and development: religion as resource. In *The Sarvodaya self-help movement*. West Hartford, CT: Kumarian Press.

Mahadevan, K. 1985: *Infant and childhood mortality in India: biosocial determinants*. New Delhi: Mittal Publications.

Manoleas, P. 1994: An outcome approach to assessing the cultural competence of MSW students. *Journal of Multicultural Social Work* 3(1), 43–57.

Mashruwala, K.G. 1958: The principle of sharing. In Kumarappa, B. (ed.), *Sarvodaya, the welfare of all*. Ahmedabad: Navajivan Publishing House.

Mathew, G. 1992: *An introduction to social case work*. Bombay: Tata Institute of Social Sciences.

Midgley, J. 1994: Social work education and social development. In Hesser, K.H. (ed.), *Social work education: state of the art*. Amsterdam: 27th Congress of the International Association of Schools of Social Work.

Mukundarao, K. 1969: Social work in India: indigenous cultural bases and the processes of modernization. *International Social Work* 12, 29–39.

Murthy, D.B.N. 1989: A new day dawns in Ralegaon Shindi. *Express Magazine* 7 May Bombay: Indian Express.

Muttagi, P.K. 1986: *Workshop on rural development: a Gandhian perspective*. Bombay: Tata Institute of Social Sciences.

Nagpaul, H. 1967: Dilemmas of social work education in India. *Indian Journal of Social Work* 28, 269–84.

Nagpaul, H. 1972: The diffusion of American social work education in India. *International Social Work* 15, 3–17.

Nahar, U.R. and Chandani, A. 1995: *Sociology of rural development*. Madras: Jaipur and New Delhi: Rawat Publications.

Nair, T.K. and Ambarasan, R.S. 1981: *Training social workers for rural development*. Waltair: Association of Schools of Social Work in India.

Patel, I. 1987: *Vivekanda's approach to social work*. Madras: Shri Ramkrishna Printing Press.

Perlman, H.H. 1957: *Social case work – a problem solving approach*. Chicago, IL: University of Chicago Press.

Ramachandran, P. 1988: Perspectives for social work training – 2000 A.D. *Indian Journal of Social Work* 49(1), 11–25.

Reddy, G.N. 1991: *The rural poor*. Allahabad: Chugh Publications.

Repetto, R. 1977: Correlates of field worker performance in the Indonesian family planning programme: a test of homophily–heterophily hypothesis. *Studies in Family Planning* 8(1), 19–21.

Rhodes, M. 1991: *Ethical dilemmas in social work practice*. London: Routledge.

Schorr, L. 1989: *Within our reach: breaking the cycle of disadvantage*. New York: Doubleday.

Shepard, M. 1987: *A report on Mahatma Gandhi's successors*. Arcata, CA: Simple Productions.

Sinha, D. 1981: *Socialisation of the Indian child*. New Delhi: Concept Publishing.

Sridharan, K.V. 1993: *One cannot step even once in the same river: a tribute to a development training centre called thread*. Samantarapur, District of Khurda, Orissa: Anubhuti Publications.

Thangavelu, V. 1978: *The Samsar model of social work practice*. Mangalore: Preeti Publications.

Thurz, D. and Vigliante, J. 1975: *Meeting human needs: an overview of nine countries*. Beverley Hills, CA: Sage.

Times of India News Service, 1996: Hazare concerned about corruption in development scheme. *Times of India* 23 February.

UNICEF 1990: *Children and women in India: a situational analysis.* New Delhi: United Nations Children's Fund.

University Grants Commission 1978: *Report of the Second Review Committee: a review of social work education in India, retrospect and prospect.* New Delhi: Government of India.

University Grants Commission, 1990: *Report of the Curriculum Development Centre in Social Work Education.* New Delhi: Government of India.

Weiner, M. 1991: *The child and the state in India: child labour and education policy in comparative perspective.* New Delhi: Oxford University Press.

Younghusband, E. 1968: *Community work and social change: a report on training for the Calouste Gulbenkian Foundation.* London: Longman.

Part 4: Contemporary issues in care

Editors' introduction

In a rapidly changing world it is offering a hostage to fortune to describe anything as 'contemporary', for 'contemporary' preoccupations soon become outdated. However, the famous saying of the French novelist and journalist, Alphonse Karr, *'Plus ça change, plus c'est la même chose'* (the more things care, the more they are the same), has some resonance for concepts of care, for many contemporary issues seem like old issues dressed in new clothes, as we see in the next three chapters.

Yet there are some issues which more closely reflect the spirit of an age. So, for example, many of the preoccupations and the context highlighted by Giarchi would certainly not have been recognizable a hundred years ago, or perhaps even a decade ago. Giarchi focuses on evidence of disadvantage among members of the European Union (EU), while stressing that the situation in greater Europe gives rise to even more concern. However, the *context* of Europe as an entity is beginning to become much more meaningful. So while, for example, community care policies have varied enormously in a highly diversified Europe, Giarchi notes that 'The rhetoric of care within the EU has been enshrined in the Social Charter' (p. 162).

Giarchi's message is rather a bleak one in suggesting that 'Discourses of power couched in the rhetoric of care justify the callous disregard for the deprived and the frail, the social and health care and welfare rejects' (p. 170). In fact, Giarchi notes how, in a remarkable challenge to traditional notions of the welfare state, market welfare systems throughout the continent of Europe are increasingly committed to privatized care. Within such systems, the scope for structured inequalities is pervasive. Giarchi points to an underclass of social care clients and health care patients whose presence makes a mockery of the rhetoric of community care. The chapter's title – 'The need for antidiscriminatory practice in Europe' – says it all.

In focusing upon 'Volunteering in a free market economy', Peelo is essentially pointing to an old issue emerging in new clothes, for the use of organized, unpaid voluntary care has had a long history. Certainly the emphasis on individualism and free market capitalism which has dominated most Western democracies over the past decade or so is at odds with the social cooperation and integration which Peelo argues underpins voluntary activity and represents diverse social values and alternative means of democratic involvement, whatever the state of social policy. Peelo notes that such alternative, sometimes gendered, vantage points are not always of interest to those who increasingly enlist the voluntary labour force to implement policies. Indeed, it is as low-cost 'care labourers' who deliver the service commodity (that is care) that volunteers are sometimes valued rather than as initiators of innovative practice engaged in expressing care which is relational and experiential. Peelo warns of the need to be aware that governments' interest in voluntary activity can be ideological and not necessarily in voluntary organizations' best interests.

Hugman concludes the book by examining the connections between community and care. Hugman does what many commentators have tended to avoid recently, namely, confronting definitions and meanings of 'care' and 'community'. He usefully reminds us, however, that some earlier theorists argued long and hard about these very concepts and, in fact, he demonstrates how the concepts have been hijacked for the use of particular interest-groups and used as an ideological gloss on social policies.

The meaning of care is identified as embracing a number of factors which need to be recognized, but Hugman stresses that 'in a divided and oppressive society ... the possibility of community care may seem to be remote (p. 199).' He argues that a more positive acceptance of diversity is crucial but that the path to that goal will not be easy. Indeed, Hugman maintains that 'The securing of equality within diversity is possibly the greatest challenge that faces any attempt to promote social justice in welfare (p. 199).' In fact, although the chapter may be about making some sense of the concepts of 'care' and 'community', the fundamental issue of reconciling diversity and equality strikes at the very heart of the social welfare debate. The challenges are daunting and the failures are dire for the future of a civilized society.

8

The need for antidiscriminatory practice in Europe

George Giacinto Giarchi

A 'culture of contentment' has emerged within a contemporary 'self-serving society' (Galbraith, 1992). Greater prosperity in the top socio-economic groups has lulled the more privileged populations in Western society into a desensitized indifference to the plight of the less fortunate deprived and oppressed people. To turn a blind eye to widespread oppression in Europe is to reinforce oppression. Proverbially, not to be part of the solution is to be part of the problem, whether the indifferent individuals or groups be in government, statutory services or in non-government or church organizations.

There are millions of disadvantaged Europeans. For example, amongst these are at least 30 million individuals in the European Union (EU) with some form of physical or learning disability (Wilson, 1996), which amounts to approximately 10–14 per cent of the adult EU population. Of great concern is the fact that at least 70% of those who are reported as disabled people are 60 years of age and over (Daunt, 1991). The situation in greater Europe gives rise to more concern (Giarchi, 1996). Given the projected increase of older populations in the European continent, the number of disabled older people is bound to rise dramatically in the next century. As this chapter will show, there are many other oppressed groups.

In addition to indifference there is also evidence of intolerance. On the basis of a major EU study in 1990, at least 28 per cent of a random weighted sample of 14 056 adults in 10 major European countries had high levels of intolerance (Ashford and Timms, 1992, pp. 14–15). As will be seen in this chapter, deprivation and oppression are exacerbated by either indirect or direct discrimination. Such discrimination is the immediate correlative of power imbalances between the indifferent higher and lower depressed socio-economic groups; between dominant men and oppressed women; between the established populations and disempowered ethnic minorities, both white and black; between the able bodied and stigmatized disabled people; and between ageist people and disadvantaged younger and marginalized older populations. The plain fact is that it is European society and its caring professions, which disables people (Illich *et al.*, 1987; Hugman, 1991).

The focus in this chapter is upon the disablement that Europe heaps upon people, not only the disabled people but also other vulnerable groups with special needs. It is European society that is handicapped – handicapped by stereotypes which have been constructed over the centuries by major institutions and which have disabled millions of people by reason of gross discrimination.

The discussion in this chapter will re-emphasize the increasing need in today's complacent society and in the caring professions for anti-discriminatory practice. Without an 'upfront' antidiscriminatory strategy of care 'quality assurance' is a deceit, a contradiction in terms. With these concerns and disparities in mind, this chapter will discuss the widespread discrimination in the European continent under the following three factors:

- Social and health care provision must necessarily be antidiscriminatory;
- The mismatch between welfare ideals and the reality of discriminatory provision fragment care in Europe;
- The empty rhetoric of community care in Europe is exposed by expediency and money-led oppressive practice.

Before considering these three interrelated negative aspects of care provision in Europe, the concept of discrimination and the meaning of antidiscriminatory practice require prior definition and clarification.

Discrimination

Discrimination is identified as societal, organizational and personal (Barnes, 1991a; Brittan and Maynard, 1984). However, as will shortly be discussed, shorthand abstract explanations often stop short of identifying and explaining the real sources of discrimination (Thompson, 1993).

Giddens (1993, p. 741) defines acts of discrimination as:

Activities that deny to the members of a particular group resources or rewards which can be obtained by others. Discrimination has to be distinguished from prejudice, although the two are quite closely associated. It can be the case that individuals who are prejudiced against others do not engage in discriminatory practices against them; conversely people may act in a discriminatory fashion even though they are not prejudiced against those subject to such discrimination.

Such discrimination is engendered within an unequal social structure. As stated by Giddens, it is not always associated with prejudice, but it is always associated with the inequity of treating some as favoured and others as disfavoured within a stratified society. Weber (1967, pp. 323–4) refers to 'dominance' within modern society, which he identifies when using the concept of *herrschaft*. Domination is effected by stratification and segregation in accordance with the old adage, 'divide and conquer'. A pecking order is set up in a society where 'interior colonisation' establishes who are discriminated against when goods either are coveted or are scarce. Discrimination is a societal European selective exercise which determines the fate of millions of Europeans who live below the threshold of decency in an affluent society (Galbraith, 1958; Room, 1995).

Social and health care provision must necessarily be antidiscriminatory

Societal discrimination is variously explained. The Old Left refers to the basic inherent social inequity of a capitalist class structure in which those who control the means of production necessarily perpetuate discrimination. The political centre prefers to posit that there are inevitable, inherent inequities within a patriarchic and hierarchic society, in which equal opportunity is thwarted by sexism, racism, ageism, disablism, mentalism, class discrimination and sectarianism. The New Right regards inequalities as reflections of human inadequacies, which in effect is blaming the victim. Ultimately, discrimination is societal in that global oppression and discrimination are woven into the fabric of the *lebensweld* (our lifeworld) in the developed countries because of structured elitism where the inequities are conserved and passed on by means of stereotypications and myths about marginalized vulnerable groups.

In addition to societal discrimination, organizational and professional discrimination are embedded within an unequal European society. Organizations reinforce socio-economic divisions, often perpetuating division by way of professionalization in formative training programmes (Hugman, 1991). In these ways separateness is constructed between the 'experts' and laity, dwarfing users, consumers, clients and patients; hence Illich's (1975) reference to the 'disenabling professions' (see also Smale, 1983). In the post-Beveridge years, during the so-called 'welfare renaissance' of the pre-1970s, passivity and dependence were often created by the professions, who not only had *power to* prescribe care, but could also exercise *power over* clients, patients or users of their services (Hugman, 1991), thus furthering oppression and increasing inequities. Given the elitism that permeates capitalism (and Europe is where capitalism first originated), it is not surprising that discrimination existed both in the heyday of the welfare state in the 1950s and in the bleak days of its eclipse in the 1990s. Discrimination is endemic to capitalist Europe, and indeed capitalism cannot exist without it.

In addition to societal and organizational discrimination, there is personal discrimination. This consists of an individual's prejudicial thoughts, false assumptions, negative feelings and biased attitudes. Although these are individualized and personalized modes of discrimination, they are embedded within the dominant European culture (Thompson, 1993, p. 20) in which everyday life is experienced. These negative means of acculturation are traceable to endemic fault lines on the social landscape of Europe which go back to the twist in the Hellenist roots of European democracy: for example, Aristotle's observation that women were 'incomplete males', the Greek concept of a male democracy (women were forbidden to vote or be engaged in the creation of a constitutional democracy), the unquestioned inbuilt 'necessity' of slave labour and the phenomenon for centuries of the 'second sex' throughout a patriarchic Europe (see Millett, 1969).

Thompson (1993, pp. 31–2) describes antidiscriminatory practice as 'an attempt to eradicate discrimination from our own practice and challenge it in the practice of others and the institutional structures in which we operate'. 'Empowerment', that perennial buzzword, cannot exist without antidiscrimination. Services are not provisions, they are in fact *what people experience*. Braye and Preston-Shoot (1995, p. 99) refer to the right of users to be treated as persons not 'cases'. They stress that practitioners should be antioppressive. The test of whether European health and social care agencies stand up to scrutiny depends on whether they pass the test of being antioppressive – otherwise they disempower the users.

There is also the prevalence of non-discrimination. By non-discrimination I mean a passive discrimination or simply an indifferent attitude towards discrimination and doing nothing to challenge it. Non-discrimination is not only not good enough, it perpetuates inequities in society, organizations, professional bodies, voluntary organizations and their staff (Thompson, 1993).

The mismatch between welfare ideals and the reality of discriminatory provision fragment care in Europe

The Commission of the European Communities' Social Charter (1989) – possibly the most significant rights-related Eurodocument to date – has deprecated 'every form of discrimination'. The Charter was adopted by the European Council of Heads of State and Government at the Strasbourg Summit on the 8th–9th December 1991, except the United Kingdom. However, it did not constitute a binding legal document. Commissioner Papandreou launched a social action programme in November beforehand to turn the articles of the formulated Charter into legal requirements. They are not yet backed by firm legislation nor by agreed agendas nor by a concerted EU shared strategy. Ideals promulgated in charters do not eliminate malpractice – they may simply provide the gloss that has more to do with a public relations sop rather than genuine public commitment. It comes as no surprise that in the Commission's White Paper on Social Policy (Flynn, 1994) there was no direct reference to care provided by social services and very little on health.

Foucault (1961) demonstrated how the most vulnerable people in a hegemonic European society have been objectified by 'dividing practices'. Foucault (1966) also identified and exposed the subtle ways in which the dominant welfare and caring professions by their interventive dominant roles reified the various states of social deprivation and sickness, turning people into 'cases'. Professional care increasingly took on the role of social policing. Also, within the *Birth of the clinic* Foucault (1973) focused attention upon the manner in which the 'medical gaze' of European professional carers and clinicians turned their patients into objects, subjecting them to treatment, in which it was assumed the users had neither say nor choice. They had been robbed of their right to self-determination within a panopticon society. From Foucault's description of the panopticon syndrome, the keepers of structured oppression, seated in high places, maintain and monitor controlling strictures to oppress further the peoples languishing below. Those set to gain by disparities also propagate and perpetuate the myth that the structure of society is necessarily unequal in which inequities and disadvantage are inevitable.

Attitudinal changes have accompanied political swings in Europe from left to right in the past 20 years. For example, in a major European survey, as many as 45 per cent of people in nine EU countries, do not support equal working rights for women and men. Also, 63 per cent do not support equal working rights for young and old and 75 per cent do not support equal working rights for immigrants. In addition, electorates have become more cynical: over half of EU citizens lack confidence in their governments (Ashford and Timms, 1992, p. 25).

The widespread introduction of 'political correctness' and of 'religious correctness' together with the EU antidiscriminatory charters are often little more than word games which cover up the malaise of structured discrimination. The problem is that the spirit of capitalism has invented an ethic to justify upper and lower levels of socio-economic groups. The 'gospel of affluence' was scripted by industrial Europe's entrepreneurial evangelists, who created the moral imperative of the 'work ethic'. Although the rhetoric of European policy pronouncements inside and outside the EU have been impressive, the reality in terms of outcome has in contrast often been self-defeating and oppressive, as the following discussions will indicate.

Disabled persons

The seminal writings of Oliver (1990), Barnes (1991a, 1991b) and Morris (1991, 1992) indicate that charters, policies and even legal sanctions have failed to eliminate widespread disabilism in Europe. Also, research designed to expose disablism has frequently been little else than discriminatory, in which the views of disabled people and their organizations have been ignored and alienated from the process of research. A UK example of this is cited by Oliver (1992) in the case of the National Disability Survey undertaken by the Office of Population Censuses and Surveys, as recorded by Martin *et al.* (1988).

Daunt (1991, pp. 6–7) outlines the rapid but uneven development after the Second World War of European legislation with regard to disability. During the welfare boom the UK Disabled Persons (Employment) Act 1944 was introduced, and three years later, in 1947, regulation regarding the placement of the less-able-bodied workforce was passed in the Netherlands. There followed a 1957 French law dealing with the need for the vocational and social rehabilitation of handicapped persons. In Luxembourg in 1959 a law was passed on the retraining of disabled persons for appropriate employment and suitable placements. Later, in 1963, in Belgium new legislation dealt with the social resettlement of the physically disabled. In Italy in 1968 it was obligatory to employ disabled persons. In Denmark in 1969, disabled children were included in the educational mainstream, which was replicated in the United Kingdom in 1970 with the Education (Handicapped Children) Act, and similarly in Italy in 1972. Although these were steps in the right direction, as Daunt (1991, p. 7) points out, the post-war measures on the whole were piecemeal in most European countries. Where they existed, they were often dictated by political and economic expediency and paternalism, which engendered an unhealthy dependency. The lead towards integrating disabled persons within society ironically was to come from outside of Europe, from California in the United States. There the notion of self-care and 'independent living' were to be introduced into Europe and to challenge 'the authority of the expert' and the professional carers.

Europe has been largely apathetic since the holocaust and the near elimination of disabled persons and has not gone far enough in supporting disabled persons. Following on from the UN International Year of Disabled People in 1981, only 19 localized action projects were set up in EU countries, with the ambitious aim of furthering the full participation of disabled people in European society. They could hardly have had a significant impact upon European society. Ironically, most universities in Europe, which are the reputed seats of wisdom, have not catered for the disabled student. It might be argued that three major macro attempts to empower the frail and disabled persons have been created: HELIOS (Handicapped People in the European Community Living Independently in an Open Society) during 1989–91; HORIZON in 1990, which catered for the employment needs of the disabled; and HELIOS II in 1993, which aimed at integrating older disabled people into society. But, as Means and Smith (1994, p. 220) point out, the impact of these and other marginal efforts was indirect, and, where they were direct, positive outcomes and improvements were modest. European government ministers for the disabled have had only limited influence, because they have usually been junior ministers (Daunt, 1991, p. 54). Also, political point scoring stood in the way of real progress; progress, for example, in the setting up in 1981 of a European action programme for the education of children with special needs was a complete failure owing to political infighting, Danish objections and German unease. It took five years before the report, 'Progress with regard to the implementation of the policy of integrating handicapped children into ordinary schools' (October 1986) was published.

On the positive side, there have been some partial gains, for example, the emergence of independent living movements, which were movements *of* disabled people rather than the paternalist agency programmes *for* the disabled and the handicapped, such as the Groupment pour l'Insertion des Personnes Handicappées Physiques in France. Also, in the 1970s, 10 per cent of the European Social Fund was diverted towards the vocational rehabilitation of disabled people. In 1975 a scheme was initiated to support housing projects for disabled people. Clearly, these paltry efforts plus the above inept measures and policies have not been very impressive.

Definitions of disability have created problems in identifying the disabled in the EU (Wilson, 1996, p. 163). There has been enormous difficulty in aggregating the various forms of disability, particularly mental and psychological disability, especially in terms of age and gender.

There have also been problems in the use of language. 'Disabled people' is preferred here in this chapter, but neither this categorization nor its equivalent terminology is used by professional carers throughout Europe (see Wilson, 1996, p. 163). Barnes (1991a, pp. 2–3) refers to the problem of agreeing about what is the more appropriate and sensitive use of language in categorizing disabled persons. The differences are partly to do with language and partly with discord over what terms are discriminatory. European dialogue between experts has halted the progress of creating a harmonized antidiscriminatory strategy. Disabled Persons International favours the term 'disability' instead of 'impairment', advocated by Harris (1971), and 'handicap' in place of 'disability', advocated by Barnes (1991a, 1991b). Direct literal translations of 'impairment' within certain countries have negative connotations but not in others. The European medical professions generally favour the usage of the term 'impairment', whereas the social services and voluntary agencies favour the use of the term 'disability'. The International Classifications of Impairments, Disabilities and Handicaps of the World Health Organizations regard 'disability' as meaning a loss of function owing to an impairment, whereas it regards 'handicap' as the negative consequence of the interaction between the disability and the environment, where the latter has failed to adapt or respond to the former. In the French language as there is no equivalent to 'disability' the substitute 'handicapped' (*handicapé*) is used by the French wherever 'disabled' appears in a European welfare or social or health care document. However 'disabled people' is the term most used by WHO professionals and is preferred by disabled people themselves (Wilson, 1996, p. 163). Nonetheless, confusions over terms and definitions persist.

Other differences have surfaced. Although technology has improved the lifestyle of so many disabled younger people it has also created heated debate between younger age-groups and between older and younger disabled persons with regard to priorities over the allocation and resourcing of the latest technological aids. In addition, there have also been divergencies and heated ethical debate over issues such as induced pregnancy termination where there has been a prognosis of congenital impairment, and assisted dying and voluntary euthanasia for very disabled persons as practised, for example, in the Netherlands (Horner *et al.*, 1993).

Daunt (1991, p. 43) also points out that the very acts of identifying people's needs and providing benefits and special caring or support arrangements have overexposed the disabled, marginalizing them. And at the same time, to 'normalize' has tended to deny the differences. As Daunt (pp. 43–4) states,

> It is absurd at one moment to proclaim that we are going to 'love the difference' and then to proceed to do everything to hide the differences away. We must beware too of those in positions of authority who may use slogans about the avoidance of discrimination and stigma as an excuse for complacency or as a convenient way of avoiding the expenditure of money and effort which practical measures aimed at solving real problems inevitably entail.

Normalization has been the in-word in the universities and care agencies in the Northern European countries including the United Kingdom, where care programmes have been initiated with some success (for example, see Blunden and Allen, 1987; O'Brien and Lyle, 1983). But Daunt (p. 44) has been less convinced of its transferability in other parts of Europe. There are those such as Wing (1988) who stress that the very suggestion that disabled persons should be normalized is 'arrogant', and implies that it is tantamount to 'welfare snobbery'. Since, however, the concept and the first programmes based upon the principle of normalization were to do with providing for people with mental health difficulties, the reason why some commentators and practitioners might share Wing's misgivings are discussed more fully in the next section.

The mentally ill and mentally impaired

The concept of normalization originated in Denmark in the late 1950s with the 1959 Mental Retardation Act, as cited by Bank-Mikkelsen (1964), which advocated establishing a way of life as 'close to normal living conditions as possible'. Care based upon the need to 'make normal' people who were mentally retarded (the early Scandinavian use of the term) was carried out in Sweden and Norway (see also Nirje, 1980). The intent was to reproduce non-disabled persons' lifestyles. The early programmes were 'equal, but separate, modes of living' in that those with learning difficulties continued to be segregated. However, the concept of normalization was to be taken over and popularized by Wolfensberger (1972, 1980) in the United States. He defined normalization as the use of 'means which are as culturally normative as possible, in order to establish and/or maintain personal behaviours and characteristics which are culturally normative as possible' (1972, p. 28).

The US model was to be imported back to Northern and parts of Western Europe in a 'valorized' and enlarged package of care. This added up to 'the creation, support and defence of valued social roles for people who are at risk of devaluation' (1983, p. 234). Inspite of the values-based approaches of both the original Scandinavian and Americanized modes of normalization, they were in effect advocating top-down, paternalist prescriptions. Imitation was the pivotal factor, but who were to be the models? Ironically, those relatively few at the bottom of the social heap, who had managed to establish for themselves satisfactory modes of self-fulfilment and their own way of life, refused to accept that normal was what so-called able-bodied people did. The many reformulations and redefinitions proposed by Wolfensberger during the period 1972–89, and his own reference to the literature about normalization/valorization as an 'ocean of rhetoric' and the implementation in practice as 'a drizzle' that was often no more than 'a frizzle' (1989, p. 184) says it all. Most of Europe did not adopt the Americanized sell-lines of normalization. Dalley (1996, pp. 100–11) in a synthetic, comprehensive critique refers to Wolfensberger's (1987) conservatism which implies that users of care services with mental impairment should model themselves upon the dominant cultural norms with no reference to alternative modes of living in terms of gender, class and ethnicity. She also refers to the moral authoritarianism that has underpinned the very prescriptive normalization approach (p. 103). Today, the way forward in analysis is away from the 'individual pathology' model and towards the societal power model, which pathologizes those who do not measure up to its contemporary, ideal, self-contained, able-bodied preferably well-heeled type. However, in the climate of a largely conservative Europe, there is increasing difficulty in politicizing social and health care issues, because politicization of discrimination issues is now dubbed as a 'radical' social guerrilla tactic. Also, the difficulty within Europe in defining key terms such as 'mental health' adds to health and social care issues.

Definitions of 'mental health' and of 'mental handicap' have been differently formulated, have created discordances and affected the interpretation of social care dialogue. For example, the German government and Belgium officials in Brussels have fought to keep the terms separate. Other European delegates have not separated them (see Daunt, 1991, p. 49). The term 'mental disability' has never been adopted by people; surprisingly, 'mental handicap' has been more common.

In Europe those with mental disorders have been the least favoured by welfare and health care law. As Swithinbank (1996, p. 78) has pointed out, European mental health policies swing from very liberal to very punitive programmes. One of the first significant European attempts to shift from professional dependency towards integration and healthy independence emerged in Trieste, Italy. There, Basaglia's influence between the 1960s and early 1980s was to lead to the 1981 Italian Act (La Repubblica) which legislated for the closure of all mental institutes in Italy (Jones and Poletti, 1985). However, as Jones and Poletti (1985), amongst others, have indicated, the benefits of the venture have been exaggerated, and positive outcomes vary within regions (Giarchi, 1996). Also, in the mid-1970s the European Commission was to set up 30 action programmes to promote the vocational rehabilitation of disabled individuals. However, results and resources were distinctly modest. Also, intransigent difficulties in identifying, numbering and categorizing the various vulnerable groups of disabled Europeans slowed down deliberations and priorities in providing care for particular categories.

With regard to mental illness, in spite of years of international debate there is little agreement as to whether and to what extent mental illnesses exist (Bateson *et al.*, 1956; Dryden and Golden, 1987; Laing and Esterson, 1964; Swithinbank, 1996). The 'regulation of the mind' has been the dominant factor in the form of tranquillizer (or 'chemical comforter') dependence in mental health programmes (Helman, 1981). Tranquillizers might also be described as mental incarceration. Elsewhere, I have presented an overview of mental health provision in Europe (Giarchi, 1996), demonstrating that inside the EU community mental health care is largely ineffective and that outside the EU mental health care is marred by historical and cultural hang-ups about the 'mad' (Leichter, 1979). It took till the 1920s before 'mental hygiene' gained a foothold in mainland Europe (Mangen, 1985, p. 8). Previously, France was the first European country to institute 'mental medicine', with its 1838 Lunacy Act. Already in 1804 under the Napoleonic Code 'the mentally incompetent were committed in a state of dementia' (see Mangen, 1985, pp. 114–47).

Also, identification of the needs of the mentally ill has been problematic. Taylor and Field (1993) refer to the ill-defined mental disorders of three overlapping populations. First, there are those suffering from one of the dementias. Second, there are those with behavioural problems, such as eating disorders and alcohol or drug and solvent abuse. Third, there are those with mental health difficulties, for example, depression or schizophrenia. Uncertainties regarding these exist amongst professionals and laity, and discriminatory attitudes and stereotypes abound.

With regard to the dementias, here there is agreement about the underlying physical disease, but the dementias are least responsive to medical care. Also, unclear notions about social and health care to deal with them are widespread. Moreover, those who are suffering from dementias are amongst Europe's more oppressed elderly populations. De Beauvoir (1977) and Minois (1989) have provided abundant evidence of discrimination suffered by older confused Europeans over the centuries – the ancient negations still survive (see also Bytheway, 1995). In fact, confusion in older people is neither inevitable nor a result *'per se'* of the ageing process; it may result from mental ill health or an unhealthy lifestyle, social neglect, multiple loss, isolation, inadequate diet, medical ill-effects within institutional settings and even medication itself (Giarchi, 1996). Wherever discrimination thrives, the victim is either blatantly blamed or aetiologies are fabricated to explain away the linkages between discriminatory practices and the social or health problem suffered by vulnerable groups. More will be said below with regard to discrimination suffered by older populations.

In spite of policies in EU countries, over the past 70 years mental health provision has been disorganized and *laissez-faire* and its definitions hotly debated. Also, antidiscriminatory mental health policies hardly existed anywhere in greater Europe. A nondiscriminatory approach persisted. In fact, European mental health policies amounted to little more than the confinement of non-conforming, marginalized citizens, regarded as 'the insane' in overlarge, isolated and dilapidated asylums.

Children

The EU has set its sights upon the dream of harmonized childcare for its 66,004,800 children up to 14 years of age (Eurostat, 1995), representing 17.8 per cent of the population. The welfare challenge is formidable and thwarted by several factors, as will shortly be discussed. Outside of the EU, in greater Europe, the difficulties facing social planners and caring agencies are greater still, in highly diversified settings, where the overall proportion of children aged 0–14 years is much greater than in the EU, standing at 23.0 per cent (see Eurostat, 1995). The children of ethnic groups are particularly vulnerable throughout the EU states and greater Europe, but research here is sadly lacking. Could this be perhaps because of a 'tell-tale' disregard for the difficulties facing such marginalized black and ethnic white minority families?

European policy statements and legislative norms regarding childcare practice, such as those provided by Munday (1992), Munday and Ely (1996) and Cannan *et al.* (1992), and the background information by Brauns and Kramer (1986), generally convey the high regard EU and other European governments officially have for the care of children, but mainly in the area of physical neglect. Also, the EU's social care regulations amount to no more than 'recommendations'. The plain fact is that the EU is primarily concerned with functional matters that are related to the organization and prioritized operation of the market and labour, so that the provision of crèche facilities are primarily designed to support the labour market 'so that parents may work', but, as we shall see shortly, even these are minimal.

The opportunities to support working mothers are meagre. There are the Community Initiative, New Opportunities for Women, and the Women's Local Employment Initiatives, but little else of consequence.

Returning to the children, the EU statutory provision of day care for pre-school children, according to the European Commission Childcare Network (1990), is scant, except in Denmark, Belgium and France. Provision is worst in Portugal and the United Kingdom. However, in the case of the three countries which do provide childcare, there are only limited places. Most children under 3 years of age are deprived – at least four out of every five. David (1993) refers to the very uneven provision for the 3–6 year olds.

Ironically, in the former East Germany many of the pre-school facilities and centres have been removed. Before the Berlin Wall was removed almost all children under one year of age were catered for by kindergartens or crèches.

According to Madge and Attridge (1996, p. 154), out-of-school or after-school clubs are even less well resourced in most EU countries. Some 9 out of 10 children have no such state-run facilities. Of those four countries which do provide for the 10–14 year olds, Denmark provides the most, whereas Spain, Greece and Ireland provide far less.

Real protection of European children from physical and sexual abuse is sadly lacking in most European countries. The problem has not been taken up as a major European issue and for the most part remains a taboo subject. The International Society for the Prevention of Child Abuse and Neglect, as cited in Armstrong and Hollows (1991), provides limited empirical sources from which data can be collated regarding childcare protection. Cannan *et al.* (1992, p. 77) refer to the gap in comprehensive data on the relative incidence of the problem of child abuse in Europe. This most oppressive and psychologically devastating area of concern is shrouded in a guilty silence in most of Europe.

Although the Council of Europe (which monitors the development of family law) does recommend child protection measures with regard to neglect, deprivation of affection, physical injury, emotional and cognitive abuse, it does not mention sexual abuse. The European rhetoric of family care sits uneasily beside the ugly face of child abuse, particularly that of sexual child abuse. Swithinbank (1996, p. 77) states that there is no Europe-wide definition of either child neglect or abuse. In fact, what is criminal in one country is acceptable behaviour in another. The 1996 paedophile sex ring in Belgium revealed the extent of well-organized child sex abuse.

Disparities abound because there are diverse laws on marriage, divorce, rights of parents and children, adoption, as well as of custody. There is no unified European policy for families and children.

Also, cultural tensions exist between the interpretation of international charters and regional or national policies, not to mention the multiple domestic cultures of care within diverse European family structures and the myriad alternative 'mores' cosseted beneath the 'crazy quilt of care'. Amongst EU states and the non-government organizations of Europe knowledge of and the legal will to deal with the various forms of child abuse are generally meagre. In the absence of a unified approach and standard legislation, in 1992 the Council of Europe formulated a series of guidelines concerned with child abuse, and advocated a much needed harmonization of child protection measures. With the exception of the 1991 Child Care Act (in Ireland and the 1989 Children Act in the United Kingdom), the abuse of children is largely swept under the proverbial household carpet. For example, there are no mandatory reporting child abuse laws nor child abuse registers in Germany (Landwehr and Wolff, 1992). Parent-centred approaches rather than child-centred familial attitudes disadvantage abused children and discriminate against their rights. For example, in the Netherlands child abuse is dealt with by means of a 'confidential doctor service', where only 5 out of approximately 1730 cases have been reported to the authorities to enter into legal procedures (Findlay, 1987; Moss, 1988). In Italy, little information is available with regard to cases that might be dealt with by the 2277 family advisory bureaux (Fasolo, 1992) and professionals tend to 'avert their eyes' when they suspect sexual abuse because of the dread of legal proceedings that must be complied with in the criminal courts (see Armstrong and Hollows, 1991, p. 153). In Belgium, measures taken by the juvenile courts to act on behalf of minors at risk are hampered by inadequate legislation (Armstrong and Hollows, 1991, p. 148). In France, although a *Juge des enfants* deals with abuse in each *département*, the judge is not obliged to see the child nor has the child the right to be counselled by a lawyer. In Spain, the child abuse rules vary according to the regional *Comunidades Autónomas* (Casado, 1992). In both Spain and Portugal an SOS system enables people to report child abuse to the authorities, but the highly sensitive and protective girdle of family secrecy hampers the system. In Greece, 'protection' is concerned mainly with socio-economic measures (Sokoly, 1992) and where in any case physical punishment of children is not stigmatized and only serious injuries are usually dealt with (Cohn, 1975; Papatheophilou, 1989; Armstrong and Hollows, 1991). Some may well feel uneasy about the EU permitting children aged 13–15 years to work for up to 12 hours in a week (The Commission of the European Communities, 1994). On the positive side, there is the draft European Charter on the Rights of the Child (July, 1992), compiled by the European Parliament (see Madge and Attridge, 1996; 130).

Sexual abuse continues to be a taboo subject in most of Europe, indeed the Council of Europe does not concern itself with child sexual abuse (see Armstrong and Hollows, 1991). Parental status is especially dominant in the Mediterranean countries, supported by 'theologies of the holy family' and in many instances by unassailable legal familial protection and domestic secrecy. For example, '*la famiglia*' reigns supreme and is a formidable normative force within the Italian political arena. In the more Latin countries, children (and their mothers) are traditionally owned by the male head of the household, in cultures where familist ideologies and possessive individualism conserve familial confidentiality. In these countries children matter, but do they matter in their own right?

The voices of children in European families are not heard sufficiently. In Europe there is a continuing tension between the rights of children and the rights of their parents. The balance is generally tipped in favour of the parents – only in Sweden, Norway, Denmark, Finland and Austria is it illegal to smack children. Exploitation of child labour is also evident in certain countries – children of migrant workers are exploited by employers in Portugal, Greece and parts of Italy and in Northern Europe (Armstrong and Hollows, 1991, p. 146).

In response to the increasing problems facing children, telephone helplines have been opened up in the EU countries. In Germany there is the BAG (*Bundesarbeitgemeinschaft Kinder-und-Jugendtelefon*), in Italy there is the TA (*Telefono Azzuro*), in the Netherlands the *Kindertelefoon*, in Ireland there is the *ISPCC Childline*, in Denmark the *Børnetelefonen*, in Spain the *Nuestro Teléfon*, the *SOS Criana in Portugal* and in the United Kingdom there is the *Childline*. However, most callers are girls and not surprisingly most are over 11 years of age (see Madge and Attridge, 1996, p. 155). Judging by the available evidence, boys and those girls under 11 years old appear to be the silent victims.

Youth

Younger Europeans may be caught up in the global youth culture, which Therborn (1995, p. 250) refers to as an 'international – largely global – generational culture'. Therborn adds, however, that it is fragmented by class, gender and ethnicity. And Müller and Otto (1986) refer to the disparities in social justice suffered by Europe's youths. Behind the glitter of an Americanized European culture sustained by a glitzy US music market is the sad face of unemployed or exploited youth inside and outside the EU. The real situation facing younger people in Europe is best illustrated by the facts of unemployment and underemployment among the young, and the specious training programmes.

Chisholm (1992, p. 126) refers to the changing social conditions of European youth, especially in Western and Northwestern Europe since the 1950s. Their schooling and training have increased, but their labour-force participation has dropped. With this, so has their income. And when they reach the promised land of paid employment significant numbers are cast into the wilderness of either serial short-term badly paid work or long-term unemployment. In the Netherlands, Ireland and the United Kingdom significant numbers of youth are on temporary contracts; in Denmark approximately 31 per cent are in part-time work and higher proportions in southern Italy, Portugal, the former German Democratic Republic and Greece (see also Chisholm, 1992). In the late 1980s the proportion of young Spanish unemployed varied from 33 per cent in Castile–La Mancha to 63 per cent in País Vasco.

The community initiative, *Youthstart* guaranteed that any person under 20 years of age would be given either some type of education or training or access to full-time employment. The 'either/or' phraseology is the nub; the fact is that many are trained, but few are chosen for the long-term employment younger Europeans require. In fact, upon completion of training courses large numbers are frustrated all the more when work is not available. Only in France is there an equitable arrangement, where the placement of trainees and job security go together. The problem is that relatively few enter the scheme, and recently schemes have contracted.

The young are also subject to highly selective education tracks. The training options may appear to be more democratic, but according to Jeffcutt (1989) they disguise inequalities. Significant numbers of highly skilled graduates, who are fortunate in finding employment, carry the burden of student loans in a Europe where once the state carried the burden. In addition, Chisholm (1992, p. 141) refers to the bitter memories of the uprisings in the 1980s in the inner cities, the recent return of the French student riots and Eastern European unrest as potential explosive reactions to society's indifference towards the socio-economic and political costs younger people have had to endure.

Only in the Netherlands, France and Belgium are there youth representative councils to voice their needs locally (Madge and Attridge, 1996, p. 156). Portugal, Italy and Germany are in the process of considering such centres.

Older people

The United Nations *Principles for Older Persons*, as cited by Laczko (1994, p. 57), states that 'Older persons should be treated fairly regardless of age, gender, ethnic background, disability or other status, and be valued independently of their economic contribution'. However, ageism has a long European history (De Beauvoir, 1977; Minois, 1989). Wherever there is ageism there is also discrimination. Negative, discriminatory stereotypes perpetuate structured dependency and inequalities in 'old age' and bolster the process of social exclusion and marginalization. Both inside and outside the EU, discrimination against older, especially frailer-retired people, very often goes unchecked in spite of well-designed policies, charters and professional codes of practice. Indeed, one might add that, because of these very declarations, real headway is blocked because the charters, mission statements and welfare manifestos are frequently little else than political veneers that cover up the real failings of Europe to care for its many millions of older people. The cultural difficulties and the organizational problems of care are also hyped to cover the main concern of governments, which is about costs. Ageism and monetarism are happy bedfellows. The 'paradox of complex mundaneity', which Baldock and Ely (1996, pp. 202–3) refer to, or *la complexité quotidienne* French planners refer to, consists, they say, of cultural, organizational and economic complexities which taken together create difficulties in provision of home care. However, it is the economics of home care which create the major organizational and cultural difficulties. Home care complexity is not a causal factor, it is an effect factor, which, with the exception of the situation in Denmark, has been created by European monetarist policies. The multiplication of assessment forms and mega-information systems, which are dictated by internal health and welfare markets and not by needs, the introduction of providers of services and care managers who purchase them, often within the same service, the intrusive and often insensitive means testing of the older person for whole, part or no payment and the mix of services who do not speak the same language and are passing the proverbial buck with costs onto allied services are but a few of the factors that create complexity, not because of organizational, emotional and economic complexities but because a money-led customer culture reigns supreme and creates the organizational, emotional and economic vicious circle which closes in upon and chokes older people's solace and equanimity. Elsewhere (Giarchi, 1996) I have explored such complexities in 29 European countries.

Walker and Maltby (1997: pp. 18–19) refer to the older people in the Eurobarometer Survey who had been 'treated as second-class citizens' in the twelve EU countries. Although the authors refer to the majority who were treated with respect, there were significant proportions who referred to a cross-section of society who were patronising and adopted demeaning attitudes towards them. The proportions of complainants and the identified culprits who treated them as second-class citizens were as follows: 19 per cent referred to politicians and local authorities; 18 per cent referred to welfare/pension agencies; 16 per cent referred to the media; 13 per cent referred to doctors and the health services, transport staff and shopkeepers; 10 per cent to the post offices, banks and financial institutions; 8 per cent to their own families and 6 per cent to solicitors and lawyers. What was missing was the percentages of those who were women, and how many of the sample were either black or belonged to a white ethnic minority group. It is these factors which are so often excluded from such questions concerning discrimination. Also, surveys are not as effective in picking up discrimination and possible abuse unless they are backed up by sub-samples of in-depth interviews which focus on modes of discrimination.

'Indifference' to the needs of older Europeans is a common form of indirect discrimination. It is a subtle form of non-discrimination. Society renders older people invisible by shifting the focus of social and welfare reform and provision onto children and younger clients, who as client-groups enjoy a higher status. They are 'yet to run' in contrast to 'also ran' populations, who are stereotyped by society as 'ga ga' and 'past it', the latter term embracing everything from remembering things to enjoying sex (Bytheway, 1995).

Direct discrimination exists within those European families who admit older parents to homes 'for their own good' in a bid to shelve responsibility towards them. We will never know the extent of the 'dumping' of older people in institutions. In Scandinavia, higher numbers (up to 10 per cent) have been placed in nursing and residential homes, which were high on the agenda until government costs proved too much and community care appeared to be a cheaper option. Justification of the sea change in Scandinavian policy was backed by the convenient argument that keeping people in the community was good practice. Indeed, it had been argued that it was so for decades in Eastern, Central and Southern Europe because families were able to provide an expedient ready-made pool of carers. In the former Eastern European bloc countries relatively few older people were committed to institutional care; most were cared for at home. Those who were cared for in institutions were placed in Dickensian, large, barrack-like homes which provided not only for older Europeans, but also for people with mental health difficulties and very disabled people; these establishments still remain (Laczko, 1994; Giarchi, 1996). What is clear is that money-led considerations have dictated trends and swings in policies.

Vincent (1995), Taylor and Field (1993) and Smaje (1995) show that there is a strong relationship between access to care and income. More will be said about the implications for care in the next section. Suffice it, here, to refer to several significant factors. First, the succession of antipoverty research programmes (Room, 1995) from 1975 to date has not resulted in a truly successful demise of widespread poverty (Room *et al.*, 1989). Second, the gap between those at the bottom of the heap and the comfortable people in the middle and at the top of the socio-economic pile has increased significantly. Hills' (1995, pp. 22–8) update of the gross class disparities in Europe reveals that little has changed since the 1970s and 1980s. Backed by centuries of ageism and patriarchy, discrimination has been thoroughly institutionalized, as also has structured dependancy.

The rhetoric of care within the EU has been enshrined in the Social Charter of Fundamental Social Rights (1989). Clauses 24 and 25 of the Charter adopted on 8–9 December, 1989, refer in the following terms to the needs of older Europeans and the necessary provision to meet these needs:

> According to the arrangements applying in each country: every worker of the European community must, at the time of retirement, be able to enjoy resources affording him or her a decent standard of living. Any person who has reached retirement age but who is not entitled to a pension or does not have other means of subsistence, must be entitled to sufficient resources and to medical and social assistance specifically suited to his [sic] needs.

However, the two 'must' clauses and the idealism that surrounds the lofty sentiments of the charter are not backed by any legal requirements, which I have alluded to earlier.

Also, in spite of the moral imperatives of the Charter of Fundamental Social Rights (1989) and its stress upon an adequate retirement income, increasing numbers of older Europeans cannot afford adequate health care nor social care.

The situation in the countries outside the European core, particularly in Eastern Europe, Byelorussia, and the Baltic countries is especially adverse for the vulnerable retired populations. They simply cannot buy in social or health care. Here the welfare rhetoric and the injunctions regarding care and procedures have had a hollow ring (Giarchi, 1996), but welfare is not given a high priority by governments of countries struggling to reorganize their economic infrastructures after the collapse of communism. Monetarism has taken over the tenets of socialism. During the early 1990s about half of the pensioners in Hungary were below the subsistence minimum (Ferge, 1992). In Poland the real value of pensioners' savings dropped by 75 per cent (Laczko, 1994, p. 26). In Romania 46 per cent of older people have been in the lowest income category. In Bulgaria the pension in 1992 was about half of the social minimum. Moreover, in the anarchic market maelstrom (see Giarchi, 1996) into which older people have been thrust, the respective states have been grossly indifferent to their plight.

In the former Eastern European bloc countries, women are generally worse off than they were under the totalitarian welfare state. The anarchy of a market economy has taken over. The question is, for how long can the peoples of the former USSR endure the socio-economic hazards of market welfare? Most are unable to pay for social and health care. In Hungary and the former Czechoslovakia, women's average pension, when the Eastern bloc countries became independent, was approximately 70 per cent lower than that of men. In Hungary, the average pension for women in the late 1980s was approximately 70–74 per cent of the average pension for men. Indeed, about 300 000 Hungarian older women had no pension at all before or after the revolution. Within the second economy, women are unable to take on the better paid jobs in the second economy. To earn enough to pay for social and health care within the new market welfare structures is impossible for large numbers of European women.

The decline in living wages of the lower socio-economic groups within the poorer countries inside and outside the EU (see Hills, 1995), upon which future pensions are dependent, the failure to index pensions with the rate of earnings in most of Europe, the total lack of benefits and state welfare assistance for millions of people in Eastern and Central Europe (see Laczko, 1994), within anarchic market systems (Giarchi, 1996), have created cultures of callous discrimination for the older generations of today and succeeding generations of retired Europeans. Ageism continues to be the unrecognized discrimination (Bytheway, 1995; McEwen, 1990) throughout Europe (Giarchi, 1996). It is fashionable for many contemporary commentators to play down the possible dire consequences of the complex conjunction of several critical factors such as: the demographic bulge of older people and consequent rise in demand for social and health care; the deregulation of state welfare and the dismantled universal care system; lower taxation and the burden of payment of care passed onto millions of older European patients, clients and users of services; the serial marriages and temporal partnerships and the resultant complexities about whose responsibility it is to care for the older kin; the escalation of costs of more and more specialist modes of care and the temporal nature of employment, which carries with it complex, fragile, transferable pension schemes and the demise of state pensions. Denial and flight from the realities, and burying one's head in the sands of false, futurist, hopes and at times even genetic-engineering fantasies, in effect constitute a type of non-discrimination in the face of the structured inequalities and hazards outlined above. Only a realist can provide for the future – the odds are stacked against Europe's poorest older populations – the majority of contemporary Europeans might not be poor (see Walker and Maltby, 1997), but significant numbers are, and for how long will European economies sustain the comfortable older majority? Unless the dangers be stressed, non-discrimination will blind us to the reality. Discrimination is rife now, as summed up by the 1993 report of the Carnegie United Kingdom Trust, *The Continuing Challenge*:

> The existence of widespread and unjustified discrimination against older people on grounds of their age . . . had been identified by the Inquiry as one of its major concerns and it followed that the programme would need to tackle the issue as a principal objective (p. 16).

Black and minority white ethnic peoples

Almost all texts on older Europeans are colour-blind. In a sense their omission is an example of academic non-discrimination. Most authors speak of Europe as if it were a white EU in a white European continent and not enriched by Afro-Caribbean, Indian, Pakistan and African older people. Most of these are residents and over two generations of black ethnic peoples and of white minority grandchildren are citizens, and amongst the latter many have adopted the host country's nationality. Although the older population has been resident for over 30 years, its cultural and social care needs are basically different from that of the host population.

Indifference towards the needs of older black and also ethnic white minorities in Europe is widespread (Giarchi, 1996; Smaje, 1995). Also, equal treatment for so many ethnic groups, especially older 'foreigners' ('incomers' is a preferable term) is not easily accomplished in a racist Europe whose affluent urban centres are attracting millions of incomers and subsequently their families. There are 11.6 million non-EU citizens (Eurostat, 1995) in the 15 EU countries plus Norway, Switzerland and Liechtenstein, not to mention the immigrant populations' offspring who have attained citizenship within these 18 countries since the Second World War. Eurostat (1995, p. 178) indicates that of the extra-EU incomers the two major ethnic groups amount to 25.7 per cent from Africa and 15.9 per cent from Asia. The Eurostat data also indicate that approximately 73 per cent of the extra-EU black and white incomers are living in three countries: about 5 million in Germany, approximately 2.3 million in France; and approximately 1.3 million in the United Kingdom. Almost a million of the non-EU citizens in 1993 were aged 55 years plus (Eurostat, 1995, p. 178) – in Germany there are 366 600 such people in that age-group.

Europe is not only multicultural, its multiple sins against humanity have built up its wealth over the centuries on the back of the mainly black slave trade. Today, the exploitation of black and ethnic white minority groups continues in the United Kingdom and the European heartland. Contemporary Europe has not shaken off the racism that has dogged its shameful slave history – scarcely any country in greater Europe has had a clean ethnic record. Racism is endemic within Europe. A leader in the *Economist* (1991) under the subtitle 'My tribe, right or wrong?' refers to the European tribalism against Jews or other migrant white ethnic minorities or black immigrants and/or refugees in West Germany, Austria, Switzerland, Denmark and France. During the Thatcher campaign the Conservative Party jibed the Labour Party with the taunt, 'You say he's black; we say he's British'. One implication of this is that the two don't mix. Being black and British, or European and black are not regarded as a rich mix, but deemed to be antipathetic social burdens supported by stereotypes, described by some authors as 'jeopardies'. For example, Norman (1985) coined the phrase 'triple jeopardy'. Adopting her terminology and substantive argumentation, it could be said that the experience of being a woman in contemporary European society is painful enough; the experience of being a black woman is more painful still; the experience of being a black, older woman is the most painful state of all! Also, in Germany, the richest and most affluent economic centre within the very heart of the EU, black and white ethnic incomers, however long in residence, do not enjoy the same inscribed rights as their German-born neighbours. In Germany, as in the United Kingdom, black immigrant families wear their passports on their faces and white minorities continue to be the butt of, for example, the Irish or EU joke. Cultural frontiers give the lie to an EU *sans frontiers*.

Lest we forget, the post-war unity of the former Yugoslavia ostensibly brought about closer links between highly diversified ethnic and religious groups and even joint ecumenical religious worship, but they were to be followed in some regions by ethnic cleansing and some of the most atrocious acts of butchery in modern times. Europe carries the long-term scars of discrimination, but a complacent Europe lulled into indifference by the 'culture of contentment' (Galbraith, 1992) has a short memory, hence it has slumbered on its comfortable perch on the fence of non-discrimination. But, when it comes to discrimination, there is no such thing as neutrality. If the health care professionals, the social work staff and the non-government care agencies are not with the antidiscriminators, they stand against them alongside oppressive discriminators.

Rural disadvantage

Large numbers of rural European people are discriminated against because of the preference given to urban electorates. As a consequence, a shortfall has resulted in rural services, affordable housing, welfare services, health, chemist shops, social service facilities and information centres, setting the scene for increasing rural deprivation throughout the European countryside (see Giarchi, 1990, 1996; Howe, 1993). The situation is worst in the former Eastern bloc countries and in southern nation-states. The factor of 'distance decay' means that community nurses, doctors, social workers and voluntary workers must travel miles to reach people in extreme need.

These drawbacks, the indifference to the needs of vulnerable rural groups with special needs and consequent discrimination persist, in spite of the efforts of such bodies as the European Countryside Campaign initiated by the Council of Europe, the European Commission report of 1988 on *The future of rural society*, the EU's Social Fund and its Regional Fund, its local rural development scheme, the Local Employment Development Action programme (LEDA) and the European Council for the Village and Small Town (ECOVAST), which is increasingly addressing rural disadvantage in Eastern and Central European countrysides.

In diagnosing the blight of discrimination, which hampers the various modes of formal care and welfare, it is necessary now to locate the underlying monetarism, which constitutes, I believe, a canker embedded within the body politic of most European countries. It is, I argue, the major significant factor in undermining the provision of comprehensive and effective modes of care in Europe.

The empty rhetoric of community care in Europe is exposed by expediency and money-led oppressive practice

First, what is meant by 'community care'? The UK White Paper (1989, p. 9) answers the question as follows:

> Community care means providing the right level of intervention and support to enable people to achieve maximum independence and control over their own lives. For this aim to become a reality, the development of a wide range of services provided in a variety of settings is essential. These services form part of a spectrum of care, ranging from domiciliary support provided to people in their own homes, strengthened by the availability of respite care and day care for those with more intensive care needs, through sheltered housing, group homes and hostels where increasing levels of care are available, to residential care and nursing homes and long-stay hospital care for those for whom other forms of care are no longer enough.

Community care policies have varied in a highly diversified Europe. They have been generated within four possible welfare systems, in which some attempts at community care have floundered and in which others have flourished. The four contexts in which community care has been thwarted or abused in Europe are:

- the paternalistic setting and arrangements;
- the synchronic setting and arrangements;
- the asynchronic setting and arrangements; and
- the anarchic setting and arrangements.

Paternalistic systems of care and welfare assistance

First, paternalistic welfare is where the state and the professions are dominant and take over welfare assets, health and social care and resources, placing them under their ownership and extensive control. Paternalism may turn despotic and a welfare dogmatism may create an oppressive anomic system, such as in the former Eastern Marxist–Leninist regimes, where the paternalism of the state was totalitarian, with the government claiming to be the all-provider. However, in practice the former Eastern European bloc states relied upon thousands of women to provide care for disabled adults and for older people unable to cope on their own (see Giarchi, 1996; Laczko, 1994). Formal provision was strong on rhetoric and weak on provision, leaving the informal carers to respond to the everyday social care needs of households in the former Czechoslovakia, Bulgaria, Poland, Albania, Hungary, Romania and Finland. Here, care 'by the community' was all-pervasive and all-important. In contrast, the government's formal 'care in the community' provision was a sham.

In the euphoria of liberation from the Nazis in post-war Europe, universalist and socialist systems emerged in several countries within Western and Northern Europe. These were tempered by the democratic values of a liberal civil society, which Esping-Andersen (1990) would describe as 'social-democratic regimes'. However, these were to lapse into being paternalistic. In spite of the intent to create a more equal society, top-heavy legal rational regulatory systems created bureaucratized care and set up production-line modes of service delivery in which voluntary community care and informal domestic care did not enjoy the same status as state-provided and formal domiciliary care (see Giarchi, 1996). Ironically, especially in the United Kingdom, the middle classes were to benefit more from welfare institutions and health care than were the working classes. In the social-democratic regimes, even the vocabulary of welfare information, of social care charters and of community care have adopted the middle-class discourse of the more articulate and more affluent classes.

Hugman (1991, pp. 82–3), utilizing Weber's concept of 'social closure' has also shown how the professions in western-type agencies have often lapsed into being structured power units, hell-bent on excluding other caring professions and organizations and usurping their schemes and on pursuing competing in-house resources. Users of the services also tended to be passive recipients, served by a vaunted 'expert welfare elite'. Inevitably within such set-ups vulnerable groups suffered within structures, which although they were declared to be 'universalist' had the unintended consequences of increasing welfare dependency, decreasing self-reliance and discrimination.

Synchronic systems of care and welfare assistance

Synchronic provision consists of a cybernetic state-centred system of welfare, where the state carries out a coordinative or regulative role, facilitating the intervention of the other welfare sectors (Svetlik, 1992, pp. 214–15). Here the state directs the provision of care, at times purchasing care and human resources in the market from the private sector and at other times procuring care and support in the voluntary sector. In the Western European countries from the 1960s onwards there was a gradual shift from the post-war welfare state to that of 'plural welfare'. The synchronic systems of welfare have been more apparent in Northern and Western Europe, where the state has remained on its podium, from which it has tenuously held on to its lead role as welfare orchestrator. These countries were later joined in the late 1980s and early 1990s by the Nordic countries.

The former Northern European social-democratic regimes (with the exception of Denmark), have reluctantly had to cut back on formal state care provision, because of costs. Lately, they have passed the responsibility of care and the human costs of welfare onto people. People within former more social-democratic regimes are finding the shift more difficult to handle because they have been more state-reliant. Moreover, the states are said to be creating a 'plural welfare culture', but in reality they are establishing a 'market welfare culture', passing the costs of welfare onto people once described as 'users' or 'clients' but now described as 'customers'.

The stock of residential and nursing homes is contracting and a community care (sometimes referred to in mainland Europe as 'open care') philosophy has been introduced. The shift had occurred much earlier elsewhere in Europe, as far back as 1962 in France with the Pierre Larogue's strategy (Giarchi, 1996). Currently, a wide variety of community household care schemes are being established to cater for the growing numbers of older Europeans, particularly in Northern and Western Europe.

Means-testing mechanisms have been designed to sort out the solvent and the insolvent 'customers' of such schemes. The ability to pay rather than the right to welfare has become the dominant feature, with a residual state providing a safety net for the most deprived and for those below the poverty line. It is essentially a system based upon the sovereignty of individualism and the power of money which discriminates against the poor.

Asynchronic systems of care and welfare assistance

The asynchronic non-state-centred system is where the contribution of the regional or federal welfare departments operate as significant partners at local levels within polycephalic structures astride civil society, which Svetlik (1992, p. 215) describes as 'self-coordinated welfare pluralism'. This corresponds more to Esping-Andersen's (1990) 'corporatist regime'. The model here caters by preference for lateral interaction and user-led self-help systems. It thrives within the more federalist subsidiarist systems of the Central European countries of Switzerland, Austria and Germany and within the family-centred systems of Southern Europe. In effect, 'subsidiarity' means that the individual must first pay for care out of his or her own resources; if unable to do so, the immediate family has to do so; if this is not possible, the non-profit organizations step in, which include the 'public-law churches and religious communities' (see Jarré, 1991, pp. 212–3).

Here, both the principle and the burden of community care are viewed as essentially familial and not state obligations, especially in the countries of the Mediterranean basin. If the family cannot cope or where it does not exist, the local churches and voluntary agencies must first provide care. The state acts only as a last resort.

Anarchic money-led systems of care and welfare assistance

The anarchic is at the other end of the continuum of welfare and care. It is wholly money-led and engenders *laissez-faire* confusion. This is a 'state of affairs' rather than a state system. The swing to the vagaries of footloose market welfare provision in a volatile economy has created uncertainties for people in the Czech republic and Slovakia, in Hungary, Romania and Poland. However, the fear that unbridled capitalism may take over has lately seen swings back to former communist parties. The return of communist structures, however, will not benefit those in need of care. The welfare system before the fall of the Berlin Wall was jeopardized by an anarchic ponderous bureaucracy which has since been largely cast aside by anarchic monetarism. The evidence to date indicates that the latter is perceived by the majority of the poorest and most needy to be the greater evil (see Laczko, 1994).

The panacea of community care in Western Europe

The problem for most European health and social care professionals, public service personnel and voluntary agency staff is that their altruism is thwarted by monetarist discrimination. Prioritization is discrimination when it is dictated ultimately by 'the ability to pay'. In effect, community care, west of Berlin (except in Denmark) is money-led.

The rhetoric of recent antidiscriminatory social and health care policies, community operational measures and home care practices have in effect been nullified by resource-led management, where a 'customer culture' has adulterated the basic altruist notions of a humanitarian culture of care. This is best illustrated by two examples, which made a nonsense of the notion of choice when the 1990 National Health Service and Community Care Act was introduced in the United Kingdom. First, older people have been pressurized into nursing institutions, when the cost of keeping them at home has been greater than the cost of caring for them in a nursing home. 'Choice' has been the flavour of the New Right, but in practice it has gone sour for thousands of older people. Second, older people have been forced to pay for their individual packages of domiciliary care or for institutional care out of their own capital when their monies or capital value are above a set threshold, even if it has meant selling their homes to meet the costs. Many frail older people have seen the savings of a lifetime spent within two to three years to pay for residential care. In effect, they have been dispossessed by market welfare.

Social exclusion (Hill, 1995; Room, 1995) in Western Europe has inevitably created social and health care exclusion. An underclass of social care clients and health care patients makes a mockery of the rhetoric of community care.

Conclusions

On the basis of the inequalities in care cited in this chapter and the mismatch between policy and provision and rhetoric reality, antidiscriminatory strategies are vital.

The welfare state is progressively presented by the New Right political European lobbies as an obsolete obscenity in a continent where market welfare systems are increasingly committed to privatized care. The magic wand is 'choice', but for whom? Privatization is accompanied by stratification and segregation, which are maintained by structured inequalities dictated by the ability of clients to pay (the new 'Eurocustomers') for what is best or better. Structural discrimination is reflected in the social divisions of tiered systems of care dictated by money. Contemporary social and health care structures in European society, whatever their mode of service delivery, privilege some and disadvantage others. The Eurobusiness of private care and pension insurance schemes discriminate against those who cannot pay for the care packages, that is, the 'Euro-non-customers', who are referred to as 'the users', who can only have what is worst, coming as they do at the end of the queue.

Discourses of power couched in the rhetoric of care justify the callous disregard for the deprived and the frail, the social and health care and welfare rejects. Disparities in care, diminishing minimal state welfare support and unequal treatment for large numbers of lower socio-economic groups are widespread. The agencies which once were proud to 'profess' the sovereignty of valuing people, by means of respect, social justice and commitment, irrespective of sex, age, race, class, belief, physical or mental ability and level of income, are now forced to shift that sovereignty to the ability to pay and cost-effectiveness in a money-led discriminatory welfare system. Hugman (1991, p. 223) in his analysis of power in the caring professions refers to the need for a 'democratic professionalism'. It needs to be freed from being impaled on the horns of direct and indirect discrimination.

References

Armstrong, H. and Hollows, A. 1991: Responses to child abuse in the EC. In Hill, M. (ed.), *Social work and the European Community*. London: Jessica Kingsley, pp. 142–61.

Ashford, S. and Timms, N. 1992: *What Europe thinks*. Aldershot: Dartmouth.

Baldock, J. and Ely, P. 1996: Social care for elderly people in Europe: the central problem of home care. In Munday, P. and Ely, P. (eds), 'opus cit.', pp. 195–225.

Bank-Mikkelsen, N.E. 1964: 'The ideological and legal basis of Danish National Service, of the treatment, teaching and training of the mentally retarded, as well as a description of the structure of the National Service'. In Øster, J. (ed.) *Proceedings of the International Copenhagen Conference on the Scientific Study of Mental Retardation*, Copenhagen: Statens Andssvageforsog.

Barnes, C. 1991a: *Disabled people in Britain and discrimination*. London: Hurst.

Barnes, C. 1991b: *Institutional discrimination against disabled people: a case for legislation*. London: British Council of Organizations for Disabled People.

Bateson, G., Jackson, D., Haley, L. and Weakland, J. 1956: Towards a theory of schizophrenia. *Behavioural Science*, pp. 251–64.

Blunden, R. and Allen, D. 1987: *Facing the challenge: an ordinary life for people with learning difficulties and challenging behaviours*. London: The King's Fund.

Brauns, H. and Kramer, D. (eds) 1986: *Social work education in Europe*, Mainz: Eigenverlag des Deutschen Vereins für Öffentliche und Privat Fürsorge.

Braye, S. and Preston-Shoot, M. 1995: *Empowering practice in social care*. Buckingham: Open University Press.

Brittan, A. and Maynard, M. 1984: *Sexism, racism and oppression*. Oxford: Basil Blackwell.

Bytheway, B. 1995: *Ageism*. Buckingham: Open University Press.

Cannan, C., Berry, L. and Lyons, K. 1992: *Social work and Europe*. Basingstoke: Macmillan Education.

Carnegie United Kingdom Trust 1993: *The Third Age: the continuing challenge*. Dunfermline: The Carnegie United Kingdom Trust.

Casado, D. 1992: Spain. In Munday, B. (ed.), *Social services in the member states of the European Community*. Canterbury: European Institute of Social Services, pp. 2–25.

Chisholm, L. 1992: A crazy quilt: education, training and social change in Europe. In Bailey, J. (ed.), *Social Europe*. Harlow: Longman, pp. 123–46.

Cohn, R. 1975: *Von der Psychoanalyse zur themenzenttrierten Interaktion*. Stuttgart.

Commission of the European Communities 1985: *The future of rural society*. Brussels: Commission of the European Communities.

Commission of the European Communities 1989: The charter of fundamental social rights. *Eurolink Age Bulletin*, Michigan, p. 70.

Commission of the European Communities 1994: *European social policy – a way forward for the Union*, com (1994), 33, 27-7-94; Luxembourg: Commission of the European Communities.

Dalley, G. 1996: *Ideologies of caring: rethinking community and collectivism*, London: Center for Policy on Aging.

Daunt, P. 1991: *Meeting disability: a European response*. London: Cassell.

David, T. (ed.) 1993: *Educational provision for our youngest children: European perspectives*. London: Paul Chapman.

De Beauvoir, S. 1977: *Old age*. Harmondsworth: Penguin Books.

Department of Health 1984: *Caring for people: community care in the next decade and beyond*, London: HMSO.

Dryden, W. and Golden, W. 1987: *Cognitive behavioural approaches to psychotherapy*. London: Hemisphere.

Economist 1991: My tribe, right or wrong? *Economist* 16 November, p. 10.

Esping-Andersen, G. 1990: *The three worlds of welfare capitalism*. Cambridge: Polity Press.

European Commission Childcare Network 1990: Childcare in the European Community, 1985-90. *Women in Europe*, Supplement 31. Brussels: Commission of the European Communities.

Eurostat 1995: *Demographic statistics, 1995*. Luxembourg: Statistical Office of the European Communities.

Fasolo, E. 1992: Italy. In Munday, B. (ed.), *Social services in the member states of the European Communities*. Canterbury: European Institute of Social Services, pp. 1–28.

Ferge, Z. 1992: Human resource mobilisation and social integration: in search of new balances in the great transformation. Paper presented at the International Expert Meeting, Towards a Competitive Society in Central and Eastern Europe, Finland, September.

Findlay, C. 1987: Child abuse – the Dutch response. *Practice*. 1(4), 374–81.

Flynn, P. 1994: *White paper. European social policy: a way forward for the Union*. Brussels: Directorate General V, Commission for the European Union.

Foucault, M. 1961: *Madness and civilization*. Howard, R. (trans.). London: Tavistock Publications.

Foucault, M. 1966: *The Order of things: an archaeology of human sciences*. Sheridan-Smith, A. (trans.). London: Tavistock Publications.

Foucault, M. 1973: *The birth of the clinic*. London: Tavistock Publications.

Galbraith, J.K. 1958: *The affluent society*. London: Hamish Hamilton.

Galbraith, J.K. 1992: *The culture of contentment*. London: Sinclair-Stevenson.

Giarchi, G.G. 1990: Distance decay and information deprivation: health implications for people in rural isolation. In Abbott, P. and Payne, G. (eds), *New directions in the sociology of health*. London: Falmer Press, pp. 57–69.

Giarchi, G.G. 1993: Reaching the elderly in the rural areas of the United Kingdom. In Howe, J. (ed.), *Altenpflege auf dem Lands*. Heideberg: Roland Asanger, pp. 40–71.

Giarchi, G.G. 1996: *Caring for older Europeans*. Aldershot: Arena Books.

Harris, A. 1971: *Handicapped and impaired in Great Britain*. London: HMSO.

Haynes, A.C.W. (1983): *The state of black Britain*. London: Root Books.

Helman, C. 1981: 'Tonic, fuel and food': social and symbolic aspects of the long-term use of psychotropic drugs. *Social Science and Medicine*. 15B(4), 521–33.

Hills, J. 1995: *Income and wealth*, Vols 1 and 2. York: Joseph Rowntree Foundation.

Horner, J.S., Cook, D., Fortes-Mayer, K. *et al.* 1993: *Medical ethics today*. London: BMJ.

Howe, J. (ed.) 1993: *Altenpflege auf dem Lands*. Heidelberg: Roland Asanger.

Hugman, R. 1991: *Power in caring professions*. London: Macmillan.

Illich, I. 1975: *Medical nemesis: the expropriation of health*. London: Calder and Boyars.

Illich, I., Zola, I.K., McKnight, J., Caplan, J. and Shacker, H. 1987: *Disabling professions*, reprint. London: M. Bryars.

Jarré, D. 1991: 'Subsidiarity in social services provision in Germany', pp. 211–17 in *Social Policy and Administration*. Oxford: Blackwell.

Jeffcutt, P. 1989: Education and training: beyond the Great Debate. *British Journal of Education and Work*. **2**(2), 51–9.

Jones, K. and Poletti, A. 1985: Understanding the Italian experience. *British Journal of Psychiatry* **146**, 341–7.

Laczko, F. 1994: *Older people in Eastern and Central Europe*. London: HelpAge International.

Laing, R.D. and Esterson, A. 1964: *Sanity, madness and the family*. Harmondsworth: Penguin Books.

Landwehr, R. and Wolff, R. 1992: Germany. In Munday, B. (ed.), *Social services in the member states of the European Communities*. Canterbury: European Institute of Social Services, pp. 1–43.

Leichter, H. 1979: *A Comparative approach to policy analysis: health care policy in four nations*. Cambridge: Cambridge University Press.

McEwan, E. (ed.) 1990: *The unrecognised discrimination*. London: Age Concern.

Madge, N. and Attridge, K. 1996: Children and families. In Munday, B. and Ely, P. (eds), 'opus cit.', pp. 126–61.

Mangen, S.P. 1985: *Mental health care in the EC*. London: Age Concern.

Martin, J., Meltzer, H. and Elliot, D. 1988: *The prevalence of disability among adults*. London: HMSO.

Means, R. and Smith, R. 1994: *Community care: policy and practice*. Basingstoke: Macmillan Education.

Millett, K. 1969: *Sexual politics*. London: Rupert Hart-Davis.

Minois, G. 1989: *History of old age*. Cambridge: Polity Press.

Morris, J. 1991: *Pride against prejudice: transforming attitudes to disability*. London: Women's Press.

Morris, J. 1992: Personal and political: a feminist perspective on researching physical disability. *Disability, Handicap and Society* **7**(2), 157–66.

Moss, P. 1988: *Childcare and equality of opportunity*. Consolidated report to the European Commission, Brussels.

Müller, S. and Otto, H.U. (eds) 1986: *Damit Erziehung nicht zur Strafe wird – Sozialarbeit als Konfliktschlichtung*. Bielefeld.

Munday, B. (ed.) 1992: *Social services in the member states of the European Community*. Canterbury: European Institute of Social Services.

Munday, B. and Ely, P. 1996: *Social care in Europe*, London: Prentice Hall.

National Health Service and Community Care Act 1990: *Public general acts – Elizabeth II*, chapter 19. London: The Stationery Office.

Nirje, B. 1980: The normalisation principle. In Flynn, R.J. and Nitsch, K.E. (eds), *Normalization, social integration and community services*. Baltimore, MD: University Park Press.

Norman, A. 1985: *Triple jeopardy*. London: Centre for Policy on Ageing.

O'Brien, J. and Lyle, C. 1983: *Planning spaces: a manual for anyone who helps set up human service facilities*. London: The Campaign for Mentally Handicapped People.

Oliver, M. 1990: *The politics of disablement*. Basingstoke: Macmillan Education.

Oliver, M. 1992: Changing the social relations of research production? *Disability, Handicap and Society* 7(2), 101–14.

Papatheophilou, E. 1989: Prevention and protection in Europe: Greece. In Daines, M. and Sale, A. (eds), *Child protection in Europe*, London: NSPCC.

Room, G., Berham, J. 1989: New poverty in the European Community. *Policy and Politics* 17 (2), 165–76.

Room, G. (ed.) 1995: *Beyond the threshold*. Bristol: Polity Press.

Smaje, C. 1995: *Health, 'race' and ethnicity*. London: The King's Fund Institute.

Smale, G. 1983: Can we afford not to develop social work practice? *British Journal of Social Work* 13(3), 251–64.

Sokoly, M. 1992: Greece. In Munday, B. (ed.), *Social services in the member states of the European Community*. Canterbury: European Institute of Social Services, pp. 1–19.

Svetlik, I. 1992: The future for welfare pluralism in Yugoslavia. In Deacon, B. (ed.), *The new Europe*. London: Sage, pp. 211–27.

Swithinbank, A. 1996: The European Union and social care. In Munday, B. and Ely, P. (eds), pp. 67–95.

Taylor, S. and Field, D. 1993: *Sociology of health and health care*. Oxford: Blackwell Science.

Therborn, G. 1995: *European modernity and beyond*. London: Sage.

Thompson, N. 1993: *Anti-discriminatory practice*. Basingstoke: Macmillan Education.

Tizard, J. 1994: Services and the evaluation of services. In Clarke, A.M. and Clarke, A.D.B. (eds), *Mental deficiency: the changing outlook*. London: Methuen & Co. Ltd.

Vincent, J. 1995: *Inequality and old age*. London: UCL Press.

Walker, A. and Maltby, T. 1997: *Ageing Europe*. Buckinghamshire: Open University Press.

Weber, M. 1967: *Max Weber on law in economy and society*. New York: Simon and Schuster.

Wilson, V. 1996: People with disabilities. In Munday, B. and Ely, P. (eds), *Social care in Europe*. London: Prentice-Hall, Harvester Wheatsheaf, pp. 162–94.

Wing, J.K. 1988: Lecture delivered to the Royal College of Arts in May, 1987. *Journal of the Royal College of Arts*.

Wolfensberger, W. 1972: *The principle of normalization in human services*. Toronto: National Institute on Mental Retardation.

Wolfensberger, W. 1980: The definition of normalization: update, problems, disagreements and misunderstandings. In Flynn, R.J. and Nisch, K.E. (eds), *Normalization, social integration and community services*. Baltimore, MD: University Park Press.

Wolfensberger, W. 1983: Social role valorization: a proposed new term for the principle of normalization. *Mental Retardation* 21, 234–9.

Wolfensberger, W. 1987: Values in the funding of social services. *American Journal of Mental Deficiency* 92, 142–3.

Wolfensberger, W. 1989: Self-injurious behaviour, behaviouristic responses and social role valorization: a reply to Mulick and Kedesdy. *Mental Retardation* 27, 181–4.

9

Volunteering in a free market economy

Moira Peelo

Introduction

Organized, unpaid voluntary care has long existed and post-war Britain has seen a multiplicity of organizations, self-help groups and charities established. Voluntary activity preceded and provided much of the impetus for the welfare state in Britain, and voluntary organizations have worked alongside official bodies. From 1979 onwards an excessive emphasis on individualism and free market capitalism has overlooked the extent to which providing care and support is about integration into social networks, not merely about individual choices. Free market ideology has provided a damagingly narrow framework within which the voluntary sector has been seen only as one means of implementing specific economic policies.

The post-Second-World-War political consensus which allowed the establishment of a formal welfare state in Britain was the same consensus which came under attack from free market ideologists in the 1970s and 1980s. As post-war optimism faded, so the notion of social cohesion as a by-product of the welfare state has lost ground to arguments about the expense of welfare; culminating in a free market ideology which defined social responsibility as an impediment to competitive success. So, as Hutton (1995) has argued, tax and social welfare systems are defined by free market capitalists as burdens which must be offloaded rather than as 'instruments of social cohesion and public purpose' (p. 16). Paradoxically, the Conservative ideology which fuelled the freeing of market forces in the 1980s also led to centralized control of care and attempts to utilize the voluntary sector in the battle against 'the nanny state'.

A commitment to economic policies which speed social fragmentation cannot value the networks which nurture an individual's voluntary donation of care. The narrow view taken by free market capitalists ignored the social networks which underpin voluntary activity and the impetus to social integration implied by volunteering. Moreover, such a narrow valuation turned volunteers from people who choose to donate their labour for free into 'care labourers', to be moved about and moulded according to the demands of state policies rather than retaining control over the care they choose to give. The voluntary sector provided an ideal stepping stone from state to family responsibility for a range of care. At the same time, pressure from within individual organizations, sometimes called the 'voluntary ethos', caused the expansion of activities while competing for public donations and funds to maintain their existing activities. The voluntary sector and government could, therefore, turn to each other as helpmeets but, in reality, were following quite different agendas.

Such thinking stands in stark contrast to the pre-1980s description of voluntary work as 'citizen action', which sounds a dated idea now. It has, however, a lot to recommend it, not least as a reminder that members of society have the potential to change society from *within*, and that constructive, voluntary acts are a part of the democratic process even if the underlying philosophy which drives that act is dissonant or opposed to official thinking. Seebohm had wanted the new local authority social services' departments to be a focal point within local communities, encouraging 'citizen participation' through voluntary activity, and so 'reduce the rigid distinction between the givers and takers of social services' (Seebohm Report, 1968, para 492, p. 151). Morris (1969) defined citizen action as 'action by voluntary workers' (p. 170) and although aware of shortcomings in the voluntary sector (such as volunteers' limited range of social backgrounds or the potential for not working reliably) she also saw voluntary work as an agent of social progress through individual action and through volunteers offering informed criticism to statutory bodies. This, she argues, is 'democracy in action' and offsets the 'minute influence' exerted when voting at elections through citizens actively joining in organizations and groups which influence policy and 'by humble day-to-day work as good neighbour' (p. 210). The politicization of issues related to care in recent years, through control of local finances and the centralization of a range of social decisions, has buried this notion of the active citizen constructively affecting policy by working in networks and groups within the community.

It was not the voluntary sector alone which became embroiled in the fallout from defining care as an individual, private matter. In 1985, for example, a Church of England commission's report on urban life, entitled 'Faith in the City', denounced Conservative policies for stressing individualism at the expense of social responsibility. Young (1990) describes the subsequent onslaught on this report, which included criticisms such as 'Marxist' and 'collectivist', attacks which betrayed the underlying assumption that concern for social issues is suspect and political, in a pejorative sense, where Christian concern should be with private salvation. Young describes the then Prime Minister, Margaret Thatcher, as shocked because 'she had found in it [Faith in the City] no recommendations to do with individuals and families, who were the source of all standards in society' (p. 417).

In a sense this turns all voluntary groups into pressure-groups which, traditionally, attempt to affect the political agenda and the exercise of power in favour of a particular needy group. As with 'Faith in the City', 'citizen action' became defined as pressure-group activity within an ideology which saw all dissonance as narrow political partisanship; or else voluntary work became assimilated into the machinery which implemented national policy. For, following 'citizen action', commentators became more concerned with 'partnership', which Clark (1991) has described as the 'polite characterisation of the relationship between statutory and voluntary' (p. 165). As Clark argues, what underlies this emphasis on 'partnership' is a set of issues about who is responsible for welfare. Partnership is a pleasant way of describing the trend, started in the 1970s, of utilizing the free and cheap labour of the voluntary sector to carry out national policy, which in Clark's study related to the effects of unemployment in Scotland. In Clark's view official grants and the later culture of 'purchasers and providers' threatened voluntary bodies' capacities for independent, effective action, owing to 'the cushioned chains of the remunerative fee and service contract' (p. 173).

Who should be responsible for individual care – state, family, society, community or the person concerned – is discussed by politicians and academics as a philosophical issue. But for the professional and voluntary practitioners it is a pragmatic matter of day-to-day work, of making the best of a situation in spite of structural barriers. These barriers are not problematic for politicians, for whom they are abstract concepts rather than an immediate and pressing reality. The provision of care and of personal social services to the needy through voluntary action is about expressing care by actually carrying out the supportive work. Kavanagh (1987) describes as significant the range of concerns which the Conservatives came to regard as 'high politics' and therefore matters for central government alone (pp. 285–6), while at the same time stripping away local government powers through control of spending (p. 287). As a variety of social issues became redefined as 'high politics' in the 1980s, this legitimate caring and concern for the needy, less fortunate, ill or unhappy was discussed as a matter either for individuals, to be carried out in the privacy of their homes, or for government-sponsored agencies. Yet the provision of care and support remains an integrated part of social networks, whether or not volunteers are defined by others as acting through informal neighbourliness or highly political pressure-groups,

Whatever the political rhetoric concerning the provision of care, increasingly larger numbers of people were donating some of their time and labour in some sort of voluntary activity. Those who research into the voluntary sector are faced with problems of definition, for large numbers of people give their labour freely for a variety of purposes, from conservation through to visiting the elderly, with scouting and selling goods in charity shops along the way. Humble (1982) reported an increase in volunteering compared with earlier surveys: his definition concerned unpaid actions intended to benefit someone, a group or some thing – such as the environment – outside the family (p. 4); and, according to these criteria, 44 per cent of his sample had done some voluntary work in the preceding year. When asked about frequency of volunteering, a substantial 26 per cent of Humble's sample worked one or more days a week on a regular basis (p. 11). Using the same ingredients in their definition as Humble a decade later researchers found that just over half of their sample (51 per cent) had done some voluntary work in the preceding year (Knapp *et al.*, 1995). These figures are, of course, completely at odds with the popular image of an ungiving, uncaring society which has typified the past 20 years, for instead they chart a steady rise in the donation of voluntary labour of all kinds.

Neighbourliness, community and voluntary care

The possible sources of provision of care, support and personal social services exist on a continuum: from individuals within families through to state provision, via paid professionals, with neighbours, community and voluntary organizations existing in between these two polarities. It is clear what the points on the continuum are, but the divisions between each are not as uncontentious as one might, at first, imagine. Neighbours can be like family in established communities, whereas elsewhere they represent the outside world; neighbourhood groups can be viewed as voluntary activity, which when well-organized, highly trained or publicly-funded can come close to 'professional' standards. By defining voluntary action solely according to the demands of a narrow economic framework it has become easier to overlook the variety of values embedded in unpaid care and the range of social networks thus represented.

Whatever the state of professional provision and the formal political arena have been, substantial amounts of personal support have continued to be provided for free by neighbours, relatives and volunteer workers. Because of the hidden nature of such giving, it cannot be fully quantified, and, given its private and unpaid nature, much of it has been left to women to provide. Walby (1990) has argued that the state is patriarchal as well as capitalist, that paid employment of women in the public sphere as carers has moved the locus of control of women's labour from individual patriarchs to the control of capitalist employers (ch. 7). Within the private sphere the role of carer has been ascribed to women as part of their housewife role, and Gamarnikow (1978) has described the process by which this private, wifely, role has shaped the nature of women's public paid work in nursing. But it has been stretched, in the past as well as the present, to encompass *free* provision of care for the society outside the home as well as inside, so much so that Hadow's report on education stressed the need for girls' education to reflect their civilizing role and ensure women were sufficiently organized to carry out their household tasks to allow time for 'the discharge of civic responsibilities' (Hadow Report, 1926, p. 234). This picture of unemployed women's public lives as an extra to their housewifely roles implies wealth of time and, therefore, money – a long-standing, if unhelpful, caricature of women's voluntary activities.

Historically, there is an established tradition amongst women of oiling the wheels of family and neighbourhood networks, with cooperative 'strategies' developed by women to provide for their families no matter how needy. Roberts (1986) has commented that much help and support was given between relatives within working-class families and that, although working-class women were proud of their ability to manage their household independently, they still 'all valued a system of neighbourhood support' (pp. 241–2). This neighbourhood support was, according to Ayers and Lambertz (1986), given secretly and unobtrusively, for need implied an inability in the role of household manager as well as advertising that a husband could not provide well for his family. This informal care in working-class districts could become 'public' work in a more systematic way. Parker (1988) describes the astonishing philanthropy of Catherine Wilkinson of Liverpool:

> In 1835 her own household contained, besides herself and her husband, two old women, four young women, two boys and four girls. The strictest economy permitted sufficient food of potatoes and broth and the evenings were occupied with music, games and reading aloud (p. 22).

She also had the prescience to set up a community wash-house in her own kitchen to boil laundry during a cholera outbreak in 1832.

The network of interlinking lives and obligations which take decades and generations to knit together can be destroyed in days through war, through relocation or through rehousing and building schemes. The romance of neighbourly help can be overestimated but, nonetheless, once destroyed these sources of support need to be replaced, or one must find other strategies for adjusting to new ways of living. By definition, as Morris (1969) pointed out, neighbourly action is spontaneous and is not organized, so formal neighbourhood arrangements can, by their existence, underline the lack of valuable networks rather than replace them. For those who are not party to the unspoken rules which govern particular informal networks of care, neighbourliness is an unpredictable and unreliable means of ensuring social support. It is desirable but selective and limited in what it can offer and, almost by definition, consistency in delivery of care must be required where need is greatest and access to support networks is least.

Voluntary organizations can appear, then, to be organized and controllable neighbourliness. Yet there are great variations between organizations within the voluntary sector, with some groups quite far removed from the notion of a local, neighbourhood group. Hill and Bramley

(1986), for example, distinguish between 'community care' as offered by large, formal voluntary organizations and that offered as an extension of neighbourly or family care. The former they see as being given by the better-off to the less fortunate, being closer to the care given by professionals and, like Victorian charity, can 'carry with it stigmatizing and social control connotations' (p. 134). Stewart and Stewart (1993) argue that it is slightly more complex, that 'neighbourhood care' and 'self-help' in geographical communities was pushed in the 1980s 'when it was consistent with policy objectives to reduce dependence on welfare state services' (p. 118), but it was assumed that the 'underclass' could not cope with self-help.

As well as geographical, neighbourly nuances to the word 'community' there are also intimations of social homogeneity and social cohesion. The impact of industrial urbanization on Victorian philanthropy has been well-described elsewhere (see Parker, 1988, pp. 23–4) as ensuring that geographical communities ceased to be represented by a spread of social classes, a situation with which (in Britain) we are well accustomed now. Conditions encouraged the wealthier to move to pleasanter suburbs, curtailing the tradition of visiting and caring for one's own neighbouring needy, whether ill, poor or merely lonely. As Parker argues, middle-class women in the nineteenth century tended to write letters, recorded their activities in diaries and spoke to male relatives who were likely to be politicians, authors and the like; but this did not mean that working-class women did not work philanthropically to assist each other through informal, unrecorded networks, as we have already seen with Catherine Wilkinson in Liverpool. Perhaps, as Stewart and Stewart are implying, there is still a range of unrecorded philanthropic activity of which many of us are unaware, being either uninvolved or not in need.

While women have traditionally provided private neighbourhood and family care, this work has, at the same time, been assumed to be the property of society both at home and through voluntary organizations (as Hadow's view illustrated) – to be demanded as of right, yet unvalued and unpaid at the same time. Marcuse was quite clear that markets function through exploitation and domination, and insure the class structure of society (1969, p. 21). The workplace is the central market, and 'labour' is needed insofar as we are prepared to pay for it and, by definition, we are unprepared to pay for voluntary work. Voluntary work is 'leisure' in the strict sense that volunteers are not usually paid and that, for many, it occupies some hours which fall outside paid employment. However, the recruitment and training practices, commitment and standards required can often mimic those of the world of paid work, and, although occupying the 'public' sphere, voluntary activity is a bridge between the private, domestic sphere and the public, organizational world outside, albeit non-profit-making in values.

For lack of pay is not the only definition of voluntary work, which has additional overtones of being benevolent. Definitions of 'voluntary' work, as we have seen, contain some notion of 'good', of 'goodwill' towards the purposes and people for whom the work is done which transcend assumptions of familial or professional duty. This reflects an essential element of 'care' as a highly personal giving of oneself with concern for a cause or for fellow humans, resulting in actions which should be beneficial. Care is an individual matter – given freely from person to person, or person to specific environment – without obvious material benefit to the giver but touching some wellspring of emotion within the carer as well as benefiting the receiver. Unlike formal politics, for example, volunteer care tends to be less about structural issues in society, the needs of capital and the exercise of power, and more about the practical deliverance of work to the place it is needed. But, unlike neighbourliness, voluntary work tends also to imply organized deliverance of care. Organizations, then, are in a position to promise to deliver future care, but they do so on behalf of individual volunteers whose involvement may be predicated on quite different grounds.

Labour, leisure and professional drift

While narrow, economic concerns might dictate national social policy, voluntary organizations cannot afford to be so cavalier, for people's choices of voluntary activities and their reasons for volunteering reflect volunteers' integration with constituent groups and social networks. Organizations, then, must meet the needs of different volunteers as well as those of government and client groups. On this Tyndall (1993) has commented that voluntary giving meets individuals' needs, particularly 'to have their own personal sense of purpose, to belong to a corporate entity and to make a significant individual contribution to society' (p. 24). This presents volunteer managers and managers of volunteers with a delicate line to tread to ensure that they recruit the right volunteers for that agency, retain them, yet, as Tyndall has said, to ensure that the purposes of the agency are always paramount whatever the needs of the volunteers.

But Tyndall goes on to say that, given the peculiarly institutionalized nature of Britain's voluntary sector, there is a danger that corporate organizations can become resistant to change (pp. 24–5), and volunteers may well expect to accept a long-established set of rules. So the experience of a volunteer who helps out occasionally in a local self-help group will be quite different from that of one who goes through an extended selection and training procedure and expects to give up time frequently and on a regular basis. Their expectations, involvement, commitment and notions of 'leisure' may be different, but they may not view themselves as any more or less caring. Formal voluntary organizations may, unintentionally, operate covert or indirect barriers, in other words, those activities which require personal resources (for example, the ability to commit one's own time in advance, provide appropriate referees and an ability to travel or to drive) are peopled by those who can meet these requirements.

These resources which people bring to voluntary activity cannot just be measured in material terms, for also of importance is the belief that one can take part in social activity; that it is one's society and a society which one can influence through cooperative social action. A sense of social confidence is not evenly spread throughout all sections of society. Knupfer (1947) described the phenomenon whereby, to protect themselves against further failure or frustration, those with least social status draw back from attempting even those activities in which, to an outsider, they might reasonably be expected to achieve their aims. In class terms, joining formal voluntary bodies which select, train and require regular commitment may well represent a sense of 'getting above oneself' and appear to require abilities one does not perceive oneself as possessing. A strong sense of social integration as a component of volunteering on a regular basis was a factor which Humble (1982) pointed to when explaining why the stereotype of the volunteer as a woman without children or paid employment was not true, and that 46 per cent of his sample of volunteers was male. The more hours of paid work a person does, it seems, the more likely she or he is to volunteer. According to Humble, 'One possible reason for this is that the more people work, the more they come into contact with other people and other 'networks', thus increasing the opportunities for involvement in voluntary action' (p. 8).

Stereotypes do serve the function of allowing ridicule to neutralize social impact, and even the most politically correct person feels on safe ground when laughing at 'middle-aged, middle-class women' apparently with time on their hands. By stereotyping volunteers as made up of some of society's least-valued members (that is, women past child-rearing age and without paid employment) we can, also, justify why activities which we *value* highly are least *rewarded* materially.

Although volunteers are likely to be middle-class people from managerial or professional backgrounds (Argyle, 1994; Humble, 1982; Knapp *et al.*, 1995), all sorts of people from all sorts of backgrounds can be found doing voluntary work, and different groups choose different kinds of voluntary caring. Knapp *et al.* found variations of class, age, ethnicity and gender in the patterns of who volunteers to do which activities. Black and Asian people were found to be more likely to volunteer for work visiting elderly or sick people. There were substantial differences between classes in voluntary activity: 'for certain informal, community care activities, people from lower socio-economic groups are the most likely to be involved' (p. 26). Women were more likely than men to work in health and social welfare organizations as well as working with the elderly but were less likely to volunteer for committee work or transporting goods and people (p. 26).

Although all these activities may be highly valued popularly, voluntary labour has always been viewed as threatening to professional status, for differentiating between professional and voluntary is not always easy. So, for example, the two 'semi-professions' (for a full exposition of this concept see Etzioni, 1969) of nursing and social work arose out of voluntary and philanthropic work; and Abbott and Wallace (1990) have drawn attention to training and knowledge, rather than pay, as an important element in defining professionalism in social work, commenting that the large numbers of untrained and semi-trained volunteers undertaking social service work thereby 'undermine the claims of social work to professional expertise and knowledge' (p. 16). The substantial presence of volunteers in nursing around the time of the First World War helped to convince many nurses of the need for registration, that important element in defining professionals, which led to the Nurses Registration Act (1919). Witz (1992) tells us that the presence of untrained voluntary aid detachments, organized jointly in 1909 by the British Red Cross Society and Order of St John, was experienced as disruptive and 'provoked disorder amongst the nursing hierarchy' (p. 160).

It is not surprising that such groups looked on voluntary work with disfavour, for one of the major attractions of volunteers to politicians and employers within a narrow free market ideology is that their labour is free and that they come without all the reciprocal ties and responsibilities attached to employed people. Volunteers can be fully trained and equipped, having raised funds to support their own activities. While government might value what voluntary *organizations* bring to assist statutory bodies in the field of care, *individuals* apparently volunteer for quite different reasons: for instance, for social reasons, to feel a sense of worth and to gain knowledge, skills and 'intellectual enrichment' (Knapp *et al.*, 1995, p. 14). In extending access to skills and training an organization is offering its volunteers what Knapp *et al.* have described as another important factor in volunteering, that of gathering new expertise and experience 'which might later generate career opportunities' (p. 14). In this sense, then, there is a drift to professionalism not just in standards of voluntary work but also as the lines between volunteer and professional become blurred and some voluntary activities become accredited steps on the road to professional status.

Tyndall (1993, p. 17) has described the additional pressures from within voluntary organizations to expand, professionalize and develop their work, citing Relate, Victim Support and Cruse as prime examples of groups which extended their work to accommodate kindred problems, having the most relevant experience to offer. Using Cruse as an example, he explains that such extensions of the core work offers counsellors chances to develop new expertise and access to training, and comments: 'Voluntary groups find it hard to resist these pressures. The organizations are free of statutory constraints and so are free to innovate' (p. 18) – free to innovate, to develop both at personal and at organizational levels, and free to meet the needs of the client group. For that is a vital part of voluntary care: a commitment to meeting particular needs, a sense of urgency in responding to those needs, and an emotional tie to playing a part in ensuring that needs in one's chosen area of care continue to be met in the future.

Managing the future

Commitment to ensuring future activity in a chosen area obliges voluntary organizations to focus on fund raising, especially in recent lean years. While cooperation by the voluntary sector with government need not, of itself, be undesirable, in this period national social policy reflected free market ideology which defined public social responsibility as an impediment to competition and so viewed voluntary agencies as one set of stepping stones to help take care out of the public sphere. Official grants and contracts, whether from national government, local government or via official agencies, were not necessarily designed in the best interests of voluntary organizations, volunteers or client-groups. The harnessing of voluntary labour to achieve economic goals started early; for example, Clark (1991, pp. 58–9) was quite clear in his conclusion that as early as the 1970s a government agency, the Manpower Services Commission, had 'colonized' the voluntary sector, that it had 'adapted, or usurped, voluntary action to help it implement job creation and training programmes required by national policy'.

By the late 1980s and early 1990s voluntary groups were seen by government as an integral part of implementing the new health initiative – 'Health of the nation' – which was designed to promote health and healthy lifestyles. 'Healthy alliances' between voluntary and professional groups were presented to professionals as bringing a range of advantages through voluntary-sector 'knowledge, commitment and ability to harness local volunteers and other resources. [Voluntary groups] may also have resources and capacity to undertake work which statutory bodies do not have or cannot do as well' (Department of Health, 1993, p. 41).

Although the same document stresses the innovative thinking which voluntary groups can bring to health matters, this approach was, in reality, emphasizing the 'service' aspect of voluntary organizations at the expense of their 'social movement' component. Quite simply, the attraction of voluntary bodies lay in their capacity to deliver free and cheap labour to the point of need while at the same time implementing government policy.

The central policies, meanwhile, remained narrow and divisive. Murdock (1995, p. 30) has discussed the 'Health of the nation' targets as they apply to mental health and has concluded that they are misdirected because, being too narrow, they reflect an unhelpful view of what constitutes mental health and mental illness. Much is made of bringing down the numbers of completed suicides and of the physical and psychological factors associated with depression. But, as Murdock argues, this is not enough; 'Social factors, such as employment, income, housing, gender and race, have a large role to play' (p. 30). Making policy means setting the goals according to one's own understanding of an issue, whereas a truly innovatory voluntary sector means voluntary bodies take part in defining and conceptualizing the issue – not merely implementing a policy decided by others. So Murdock points to the alternative definitions of mental health care put forward by MIND, whose targets would include social aspects of mental health care. In addition, Murdock argues that the introduction of a free market economy into the National Health Service manufactured a split between the assumed 'purchaser' and those contracted to be 'providers', a divide which hampers joint planning and coherent funding.

A part of free market ideology has been the belief that markets are always desirable, bringing competition, which automatically leads to efficiency. Hence 'internal markets' became the order of the day in the public sector, with a range of professionals – from general practitioners to head teachers – becoming 'budget holders' who could, technically, buy whatever services they needed. Internal markets had the effect of demarcating groups, separating out purchasers from providers of services. Hence a management culture and style existed which worked against cooperative systems of organization. As within the National Health Service, for example, this particular management style objectified care, making it a commodity to be bought and sold like any other consumer product. 'Objectification' of care means invalidating the emotional, experiential and relational components of care and turning it, instead, into just another service to be managed and delivered to where it is needed. The person who cares, then, becomes a labourer who must be made to deliver efficiently, economically and without emotional encumbrances (such as notions of duty, responsibility or concern for relationships). Like care itself, the emotional elements which constitute caring, giving relationships become defined as private and personal matters which may motivate individuals but which have no part in a public agenda.

The emphasis on this style of efficiency and on internal markets gave undue prominence to managers and management style, as this seemed to promise the desired outcomes within a free market economy. Based on the demands of funding, this management style separated carer and cared for by defining the nature of their relationship in terms of purchaser and provider. Whatever the intentions of the giver or the needs of the receiver, their relationship was mediated through an agent who acted as buyer of the commodity (care), so turning the carer into a purveyor of that care. In time, this management style, which objectified care, was applied to some parts of the voluntary sector. For example, the Marriage Guidance Council (now known as Relate) was having difficulty adjusting to the financial rigours of the 1980s in which, in spite of rhetoric which supported families, government grants did not match the organization's expansion (Lewis and Morgan, 1994). Lewis and Morgan show that the Marriage Guidance Council adopted a managerial solution to problems by strengthening their management structure where previously it had been their tutorial and counselling structure which had been powerful. The style of management analysis used – one of 'technical rationality' (p. 661) – entirely overlooked the nature of the organization and was a style which attempted 'to impose the business methods of the private sector on a voluntary agency' in an inappropriate way for the nature of the Marriage Guidance Council (p. 661). In an already highly gendered organization, where administration values were perceived as masculine, this approach devalued what were experienced as 'feminine', counselling values of caring and mutual support. In so doing changes appeared to crush the therapeutic values which gave the Marriage Guidance Council its value in the eyes of many of its counsellors.

In the 'Relate' example above, fragmentation was exacerbated by adopting solutions to economic crisis which devalued the organization's core values and workers. In the case of the Oxford Cyrenians, funding solutions appeared to separate the organization from its core skills, which became less relevant to the needs of a new situation which emerged out of the expansion of hostel facilities (OHA, 1995). Tragedy produces inquiries, hence exceptional events occasionally lift the curtain to reveal what it is that has become daily practice. The death of Jonathan Newby as a result of being stabbed by a hostel resident was the worst imaginable outcome of being a volunteer worker. In 1993 he was working for Oxford Cyrenians; he was poorly paid, gaining experience which can be a route either into social work or to progress within paid work in the voluntary sector. The subsequent report to Oxfordshire Health Authority charted the process by which policies of community care for a range of mental health patients meant that Oxford Cyrenians' clientele were changing, as the 'contract culture' allowed them to fill a social services void. So, rather than a focus on single homelessness and its accompanying distress (where Cyrenian expertise lay), the balance had swung to mental illness taking precedence in Jaqui Porter House where Newby finally worked, making the practices and systems which the Cyrenians had built up over years seem ineffective. The Inquiry Report recognised a 'chain of causation' (p. 141), a cocktail of particular circumstances, which led to such an unhappy outcome. Among these circumstances some stand out: agency responsibility for registering hostels, insufficient means by which to recognize and respond to the growing crisis and keeping to old, no longer appropriate, practices.

Amongst many criticisms made of Oxford Cyrenians in the inquiry was the lack of appropriate qualifications on the part of Newby's line managers. Clark (1991) also drew the conclusion that little theory was drawn on in the work of his sample of organizations responding to unemployment in Scotland. Although Clark is aware that mistakes must be made if organizations are to be innovative, his solution of carrying out more research into voluntary action is ingenuous since this must mean one researches while avoidable mistakes are made (p. 174). Ultimately, voluntary social action must impact on people who use the services provided, and carrying out evaluative research will not save them from being subject to others' mistakes. Yet one could argue that trained volunteers with a 'theory-based knowledge' are merely underpaid or unpaid social workers, and although it is not enough for volunteers to claim goodwill as a substitute for good practice, the assimilation of volunteer work into a social work worldview professionalizes care. Professionalization of care is not just about standards, financial power or ownership of certain types of knowledge (although it is all these). Rather it means that, additionally, one works in certain ways to demonstrate possession of the credentials needed to join in particular activities, which are then confirmed (or not) by professionals and government agencies.

Most people join in society at the level at which they perceive themselves to be able to contribute and to participate. While commentators (such as those we have already met: Clark, Morris, Seebohm or Wolfenden) assess the use of the voluntary sector by its perceived functions as innovatory and as a state gap-filler in provision, in fact it exists because people continue to do voluntary work. If levels of knowledge and skill required to carry out voluntary activity spiral, then one may well begin to recruit from a different pool of people, and one's usual volunteers will disperse elsewhere.

One could take Clark's argument forward and argue that by selling the labour of genuine volunteers, voluntary organizations have colluded with funders to extract professional standards while paying relatively little for the service given. Fragmentation becomes institutionalized within voluntary organizations if voluntary-sector managers begin to move away from their volunteers by virtue of the strategies developed to ensure future funding of their activities. While their vision may be great, nonetheless persuasion, consultation and debate would be necesary within organizations to ensure that volunteers move their personal vision of care too if one is to avoid the kinds of internal upheaval undergone by the emergent Relate organization in the 1980s. Perhaps the extra knowledge needed by volunteers lies less in theoretical social work and more in how to ensure that your labour is not sold by voluntary-sector managers (whether these be paid community workers, professional managers or voluntary committees) to a third party in exchange for money to fund the future of the activity.

Acknowledgements

Thanks to Brian Francis, Joan Guenault and Roger Hadley for commenting on earlier drafts of this chapter and to Ruth Wain for discussions and caravan space for writing.

References

Abbott, P. and Wallace, C. 1990: Social work and nursing: a history. In Abbott, P. and Wallace, C. (eds), *The sociology of the caring professions*. Basingstoke: Falmer Press, pp. 10–28.

Argyle, M. 1994: *The psychology of social class*. London: Routledge.

Ayers, P. and Lambertz, J. 1986: Marriage relations, money and domestic violence in working-class Liverpool, 1919–39. In Lewis, J. (ed.), *Labour and love: women's experience of home and family 1850–1940*. Oxford: Basil Blackwell, pp. 195–219.

Clark, C.L. 1991: *Theory and practice in voluntary social action.* Aldershot: Avebury/Gower.

Department of Health 1993: *Working together for better health.* London: HMSO.

Etzioni, A. 1969: *The semi-professions and their organization.* New York: The Free Press.

Gamarnikow, E. 1978: Sexual division of labour: the case of nursing. In Kuhn, A. and Wolpe, A. (eds), *Feminism and materialism.* London: Routledge and Kegan Paul, pp. 96–123.

Hadow Report 1926: *The education of the adolescent.* London: HMSO.

Hill, M. and Bramley, G. 1986: *Analysing social policy.* Oxford: Basil Blackwell.

Humble, S. 1982: *Voluntary action in the 1980s: a summary of the findings of a national survey.* Berkhamsted: The Volunteer Centre.

Hutton, W. 1995: *The state we're in.* London: Vintage Books/Random House.

Kavanagh, D. 1987: *Thatcherism and British politics: the end of consensus?* Oxford: Oxford University Press.

Knapp, M., Koutsogeorgopoulou, V. and Smith, J.D. 1995: *Who volunteers and why? The key factors which determine volunteering,* Third Series, Paper 3. London: The Volunteer Centre.

Knupfer, G. 1947: Portrait of the underdog. *Public Opinion Quarterly* **11**, 103–14.

Lewis, J. and Morgan, D. 1994: Gendering organizational change: the case of Relate, 1948–1990. *Human Relations* **47**(6), 641–663.

Marcuse, H. 1969: *An essay on liberation.* Harmondsworth: Penguin Books.

Morris, M. 1969: *Voluntary work in the welfare state.* London: Routledge and Kegan Paul.

Murdock, D. 1995: Redefining the targets for mental illness. *Nursing Standard* **9** (49), 28–30.

OHA 1995: *Inquiry into the circumstances leading to the death of Jonathan Newby (a volunteer worker) on 9th October 1993 in Oxford.* Oxford: Oxfordshire Health Authority.

Parker, J. 1988: *Women and welfare: ten Victorian women in public and social service.* London: Macmillan.

Roberts, E. 1986: Women's strategies, 1890–1940. In Lewis, J. (ed) *Labour and love: women's experience of home and family 1850–1940.* Oxford: Basil Blackwell, pp. 223–247.

Seebohm Report 1968: *Report of the Committee on Local Authority and Allied Personal Social Services.* Cmnd 3703. London: HMSO.

Stewart, G. and Stewart, J. 1993: *Social work and housing.* London: Macmillan.

Tyndall, N. 1993: *Counselling in the voluntary sector.* Buckingham: Open University Press.

Walby, S. 1990: *Theorizing patriarchy.* Oxford: Basil Blackwell.

Witz, A. 1990: *Professions and patriarchy.* London: Routledge.

Young, H. 1990: *One of us.* London: Pan.

10

Community and care

Richard Hugman

Introduction

In recent decades the terms 'community' and 'care' have become tied very closely together in the health and social welfare arena. This can take the form of an explicit reference to 'community care', as in the United Kingdom, or 'community options' for care as in the United States (McDowell *et al.*, 1990; Means and Smith, 1994). In other national contexts there is an emphasis on care 'at home', as with the French policy of *maintien à domicile* (Henrard, 1991). In Australia the two concepts have been brought together in the 1985 Home and Community Care Act and subsequent policy implementation (Ozanne, 1990). However, the common thread running through health and welfare developments across advanced industrial countries is that of a movement towards the location of care for people who require assistance in daily living within the wider structures of society and not solely within specialized institutions. In this sense all such countries have pursued policies of community care, usually staffed by professionals who, in many cases, have been the driving forces for community-based provision.

This chapter examines the connections between community and care. Given the strong connection in both policy and practice which has developed, the question of whether community and care are synonymous is considered. From this point, the issue of what else 'community' might embody, and whether this is contradictory to the idea of 'care', is explored. In conclusion, the chapter considers the implications for the concept of care in practice arising from its contemporary identification with community.

Community and the meaning of care

Social anthropologists and sociologists have argued long about the definition of 'community' (Bulmer, 1987). In a classic text, Redfield (1960) summarized the multifaceted identity of this concept, noting that its defining features include a set of close social relations, small-scale social structures, a distinctive social psychology, a shared history and outlook on life and a particular place in the larger national society; it is even a combination of opposites. The anthropological work from which Redfield and his contemporaries derived their understanding was undertaken largely in pre-industrial countries or the rural areas of those which had industrialized. To this extent his formulation misses the point of earlier sociologists whose intellectual project was founded on an analysis of the rapid social changes endemic to industrialization. Tönnies, Simmel and Le Play, as well as Durkheim, Marx and Weber, can be seen as having responded to the late nineteenth century view that 'community' was something that had been lost in the processes of rapid urbanization that followed the industrial revolution (Nisbet, 1966). Where the social anthropologists sought to describe and analyse extant (if sometimes disappearing) social forms, the sociologists had struggled to grasp that which had been lost, the emergent structures and patterns of society and to both anticipate and influence that which was to come.

More recently, the idea of community has re-emerged in policy and practice as well as in the interests of academic researchers and theorists, if (given the history of social science noted above) it can be said ever to have disappeared (Pereira, 1993). Although there continues in some lines of thought to be a sense that community describes previous social conditions, a bygone age, an approach to community also has grown which appears to take at face value certain of the features described by Redfield, especially in the sense of close social relations, shared interests and a common location for daily life. For example, the discussion of community in the Barclay Report on social work in the United Kingdom places particular emphasis on shared interests and common places of daily living as defining attributes (NISW, 1982).

Although the Barclay Report separated these elements analytically, government policies have often tended to collapse them together. In this juxtaposition of 'interests' and 'location' there is a hazard that consists of assuming a positive connection between the two. In other words, the all-purpose use of the term to embrace both attributes together, without questioning the evidence for such a position, leads to a presumption that shared locations necessarily involve shared interests. Such a conclusion ignores another facet of the anthropological tradition, that communities are also 'a combination of opposites' and are likely to be divided, even contradictory. It cannot be assumed that communities of place are united by common concerns and views of the world, nor can it be taken for granted that people who share interests live in close proximity. Yet it is just such an assumed connection which appears to lie at the heart of community care developments around the world. The idea of community has become strong on positive values but weak in relation to critical comprehension, what

Titmuss called 'the everlasting cottage-garden trailer' (quoted in Bulmer, 1987, p. 15).

Baldwin (1993) argues for the rejection of the idea of community as it has been applied to health and welfare services. From the perspective of professional services 'a community' may be large, artificially defined and relate predominantly to the organization of the professional services. In contrast, Baldwin proposes a 'neighbourhood' approach, focused on small, discrete places which relate to the lives of ordinary people. The use of the term 'community' to which Baldwin points is clearly very different from that of the social anthropologists, whose emphasis was on small-scale settings involving primary relationships and shared interests, or even from aspects of the Barclay Report, which echoed these elements although the report as a whole failed to grasp the implications of these ideas. In this sense it may be said that the concept of community has been hijacked for the use of particular interests within the professions and as an ideological gloss on social policies.

Family and community care

This ideological use of 'community' serves to support another aspect of community care policy which also has tended to be treated in an unproblematic fashion: the family. The UK government report *Growing older* (DHSS, 1982) explicitly stated that care in the community was to mean care by families, and that policy would be directed towards encouraging families to undertake this task. An Australian report of the same year came to similar conclusions, providing the basis for the subsequent Home and Community Care Act of 1985 (McLeay, 1982; Ozanne, 1990). The family, therefore, may be said to be the type of small-scale social structure which is pivotal in community care. Indeed, to the extent that community care is identified as care at home, then the family plays a central active part.

However, the feminist critique of this link between the family and caring exposes the extent to which the meaning of community is collapsed by the decisions of policy-makers and professionals (Dalley, 1988). As Finch and Groves (1980) demonstrated in an influential analysis, the family too is a contradictory set of social relations, in which not all parties are equal: care by the community not only means care by families, it means overwhelmingly care by women members of families. (For discussions of men as carers, see Arber and Gilbert, 1989; Fisher, 1994.) So even the most widespread experience of colocation and close social relations, that of shared residence in a family home, cannot be assumed necessarily to create common interests when it comes to the division of caring labour. The communities of interest shared by (most) women and (some) men around the issue of caring cut across families and other social relations.

In this way such communities of interest may serve to divide communities of place, leading to the social exclusion of some people from their locality by virtue of their caring role (Ungerson, 1990). If in being a carer one is prevented from taking part in normal social activities because of the impact of those responsibilities, this is as much a barrier to citizenship as is poverty (Roche, 1992). (That many carers experience poverty is a compounding factor in the experience of caring (Jani-le Bris, 1992).) The implication here is that membership of one community ('carers') inhibits or totally prevents participation in another (local social structures and social relations). The gendering of such communities pervades the welfare state, in which the construction of policies and practices maintains this division (Bryson, 1992). As Bryson notes, the capturing of the political agenda around welfare by economic conservatives (of all parties) has tended to reinforce this trend and to emphasize explicitly a perception of the family which previously had been implicit. (I will return to this point below.)

The meaning of care proposed by Mayeroff (1972) had certain parallels to the elements of community which have been discussed above. Mayeroff understood caring to be a combination of 'commitment' (intent to see another person develop and achieve their potential) and the intellectual and emotional characteristics of the person who is seen as caring (possession and use of knowledge and moral values). He distinguished also between commitment to a person and commitment to an idea; for example, between 'I care about you' and 'I care about social justice'. However, Mayeroff's discussion contrasts caring to the sense of 'burden' which may be experienced in performing tasks for the good of another. Elsewhere I have noted that this is a tautology, in that the person who expresses a sense of burden will be seen as 'uncaring' (Hugman, 1991). In the context of community this becomes a vital issue. Feminist critiques of community care have argued that social policies have been built on assumptions about the connections between family and commitment. Namely, that families (and hence largely women) should not experience (or at least not express) a sense of burden in performing care tasks for relatives, because these are people for whom they will (or should) feel a sense of commitment. Thus, there is a compulsion to act *as if* this sentiment is 'real'. Assumptions about connections between community of interest and community of place, which are built into community care policies, in many instances may lead to enforced caring. Compulsory altruism clearly is a *non sequitur*, yet this is the direction in which community care policies have moved (Davis and Ellis, 1995). In contrast, Ungerson (1983) has distinguished between 'caring for' and 'caring about' to represent the difference of performing tasks to feeling concern; Graham (1983) similarly separates 'labour' from 'love'. This separation provides the basis not only for recognizing that the two are distinct but also for seeing that the care of commitment does not have to be expressed through the performance of particular tasks. Caring about another, loving that person, may just as reasonably be conveyed through ensuring the tasks of caring for her or him, the labours of meeting her or his daily needs, are undertaken by appropriate professionals.

At the same time, not all feminists wish to abandon the gains which can be made through community care policies. As a disabled woman Morris (1991) argues that much of the attack on the interlocking of community and care has focused on women who do not wish to be carers. As a disabled woman who wishes to remain in her own home, Morris is concerned to defend policies (and hence services) which will enable her to do so with as much care from her partner as they together decide is appropriate. For her as a disabled woman the shared commitments and shared residence do come together. The situation faced by black and ethnic minority women may be seen as comparable in some respects. Bryan *et al.* (1985) write about feeling forced to take sides with black men against racism in ways which separate them from white women. This may mean arguing for community care services, even when they are built on assumptions about family and community. For many black and ethnic minority carers the support of relevant services simply is not available. However, this is not because the state has reconstructed care to place a greater emphasis on the family but because the needs of minority 'racial' groups largely are unrecognized (Gunaratnam, 1993).

Although disabled and black and ethnic minority defences of community care have often been constructed as at least partially oppositional to the earlier critiques, this is not to say that they accept the assumptions discussed above about connections between community and care. Frequently, it is as much a part of their critique that the community is obliged to undertake the labour of care beyond their wishes or capacities. Nor do these analysts wish to distance themselves from a feminist perspective. Rather, through noting that this debate highlights the ways in which 'disability' and 'race' may also create different communities of interest, for men as well as for women, the question of identity is brought to the fore. Community in this sense is how we define ourselves, which involves commitment and a pattern of expressing our concern for those with whom we identify. The vital element in this understanding of community, which as Morris (1991) notes reconnects with earlier feminist arguments, is that of choice. Without the sense that commitments are willingly accepted there is no community. As a disabled woman, for Morris, this means that the choice not to enter collective care but to remain in her own home with her partner must be viable.

This sense of living 'at home' draws us back to ideas about place and suggests that location is, in fact, still an important ingredient in the overall analysis of community and care. So in the next sections of this chapter I will consider negative and positive aspects of location as a central feature of community care policy and practice.

Not in an institution

Another way of understanding 'community' is by examining that which it is not. Possibly the simplest definition which can be offered in this respect is to say that the community is 'not an institution'. In this context the term 'institution' not only denotes an specific structure for the provision of care, such as a hospital, a hostel or a residential home, but also has become embedded with specific values. The use of the adjective 'institutional' is not simply descriptive but carries a pejorative tone. The origins of this view, like those of the meaning of community, may be sought in the work of a previous generation of social scientists. Chief among these was Goffman (1968) whose concept of the 'total institution' has had a major impact on subsequent cohorts of policy-makers and professionals. For Goffman, all types of institutions share certain characteristics which include: the separation of inmates [sic], literally or symbolically, from the rest of society; limits to or the denial of the individuality of inmates; the concentration of all aspects of life in one place; and the control by others of the use of time and space by inmates (who in health and welfare services are usually care staff, such as nurses, social workers and so on). This led, in Goffman's analysis, to the 'mortification of the self', the eradication of the personhood of the inmate by the pattern of institutional life.

Examples of the ways in which these factors have been seen to operate institutionally include the forcible bathing of new residents, regimented mealtimes, a lack of personal property (including clothing), a general lack of privacy (dormitories, the use of commodes or toilets without doors) and denigratory language used by staff towards residents (Hugman, 1994, p. 131). That these examples are all taken from residential health and social services for frail elderly people, and all date from the 1970s to the 1990s, underlines the currency of Goffman's observations. Observations of such conditions in health and social welfare services can be dated to the early 1950s, with increasing concern about the large mental hospitals in the United Kingdom, for example (Means and Smith, 1994). In contrast to the institution as described by Goffman, the community is understandable in terms of choice and individuality, expressed through personal control over daily life. To the extent that life outside institutions offers these possibilities, then moves 'to the community' may indeed be a positive step for the provision of services.

The historical period in which institutional care developed was that of the industrial revolution. Scull (1979) argues that just as many forms of work were taken out of the home and into the factory, so the care of people with illness or disability also were congregated on a comparable scale, in large hospitals that were the 'factories' or 'warehouses' of health and social welfare. The explanation which Scull (1984) offers for the emerging challenge to the legitimacy of these structures is not that Western industrial society has become more human, but that new technologies are being developed that make the large institutions obsolete. In contrast to Scull, Murphy (1991, quoted in Means and Smith, 1994) suggests that, *in their time*, the large institutions may have been an improvement on the quality of life experienced by people with ill health or disabilities. However, most commentators appear to be in agreement that the enthusiasm on the part of governments for community care, seen as that which is not institutional, is based on a concern with the costs of institutions compared with the perceived costs of other forms of care rather than on a concern with issues of quality or abuse (Means and Smith, 1994, p. 38).

Scull (1984) suggests we should go further and ask whether the new technologies actually represent a significant shift in social relations or whether the move out of the institution is socially acceptable only because there are now other ways of controlling the people concerned. The extent of personal choice and control is seen as limited at best and often illusory in this analysis.

In a situation of limited public funding for health and welfare programmes this may be an accurate observation. For the person living on his or her own in public housing, on very low income, and whose range of activities is defined by welfare services (the day centre, the drop-in centre, the lunch club and so on) the level of choice and control is nowhere near that of the person with a more substantial income. Moreover, the person with greater income is more likely to be involved in roles and activities which in themselves are socially valued. Indeed, it may be that these are the factors which make for a non-institutionalized lifestyle and that Goffman's concept of the total institution should be considered from this perspective. For example, the day-to-day lives of university students may share some of the features of this concept but, like the members of religious orders and crews of cargo ships discussed by Goffman, the identity of students, as that of nuns or sailors, is (for the most part) one which carries predominantly positive social value.

At the same time, however, the choice and control in their own lives exercized by university students is not unlimited. The control by nuns or sailors over their own lives is curtailed, albeit by choice. This suggests that, as measures of institutionality, such factors are highly relative. It is in this respect that advocates for service users have sought to extend the range of options available through the development of services which are as least institutional as possible (McDowell *et al.*, 1990; Warner, 1991). Warner (1991) stresses that the key factors are the availability of creative alternatives in which the opportunities for choice and control by the service user can be maximized, and the availability of funds. In many circumstances, 'the community' therefore might be a group home or other shared residential facility in preference to a large hospital. In other situations, however, it might not be seen in this way. The extent to which a residential home would be experienced as community living would, I suggest, follow from the place in which the person concerned had previously lived. For the person whose alternative location for the use of services was in a large hospital with a very restrictive regime, a residential facility of 50 people might be seen as 'in the community'. To the person currently resident in their own home the same place might appear to be an institution.

It is for this reason that there may appear to be a confusion in the language of community care. For some people, who have lived within a large institution, community care will be understood as leaving the hospital. Community in this perspective is that which is outside the institution. For other people, who require assistance to accomplish daily living, community care may be defined as not having to live within a group to receive that help. From this point of view any sense of 'the community' will be based on the ordinary living which the person has previously experienced. The type of location, the size of group with whom one lives and the overall lifestyle which constitutes 'community care' will differ between individuals, relative to their experience, their goals and ambitions and so on. Attempts to refine this understanding even more exactly therefore seem likely to continue to produce quite different claims about appropriate and acceptable patterns of services and the structures through which they are provided.

The meaning of home

Opposed to the idea of the 'total institution' may be countered the notion of 'home'. It is at home that one is able to express individuality and exercise a limited degree of choice over the use of time and space which institutionality denies. As Bulmer (1987, pp. 57–66) notes, there is a parallel in the process of the development of the home in industrial society to the emergence of the factory system of work (and, as discussed above, institutional forms of care). The separation of different parts of social life through the specialized use of spaces for work and play, as well as private family space, key elements in the 'total institution' concept, also has its origins in the historical forces of industrialism and urbanism. In this way the home as the opposite to the institution can be seen as part of a contradiction. It has been formed by the privatization of domestic space, taking it out of the community as previously understood as much as were the places of work. This has been observed by the critics of 'privatization'(Bulmer, 1987), but was unrecognized in the work of Goffman or subsequently by those who have used his ideas to reshape caring services.

A major influence in recent decades has been the principle of 'normalization' in caring services (for example, see Wolfensberger and Tullman, 1989). Although there is a great deal of debate about the precise definition of the principle it may be summarized in terms of the restructuring of services so that they promote the elements of normal life which are to be found in ordinary society (Rapley and Baldwin, 1995). The principle is in stark contrast to the total institution. On the basis of citizenship (inherent but largely unelaborated) in this work, the promotion of certain styles of living by users of caring services is highly plausible. It c in be put simply in terms of offering to others the type of lifestyle which one accepts for oneself. However, the social analysis underlying this approach was mostly unexplored (Rapley and Baldwin, 1995) nor was the debt to Goffman explicitly acknowledged (for example, see Perrin and Nirje, 1989, p. 226). As a consequence the dominant formulation of the principle tended to produce a reified concept of both 'home' and 'community'. An unfortunate outcome was that some professionals thereby turned the critique of institutions into a technical problem, one which could be resolved by mechanistic means and by treating colleagues or others who disagreed as constituting ill-intentioned resistance (Brandon, 1991). It also tended to reduce the move from large institutions to an issue of physical integration, ignoring the social dimensions of 'home' and 'community', in the relationships of which they are composed and in issues of choice. (Perrin and Nirje (1989) are particularly critical on the latter point.)

In the description by Morris (1991), discussed above, of the way in which she would wish to be cared for there is an embedded statement about the meaning of home. It can be seen as that space, controlled by Morris and her partner, in which they are able to live in such a way that their commitments (including their personal relationship) are integrated with the needs one partner has for assistance with certain aspects of daily living. A somewhat different approach to care at home is described by Macfarlane (1993), in a scheme through which two women with disabilities sought to use public funding for support services which they controlled directly (rather than through a professional as intermediary). Home for these women also is that space in which they could exercise choice and control over their daily lives and needs. Community is the wider set of *local* social structures and social relations within which home is located and by which it is supported; in other words, it is people and the activities, commitments and relationships which make up their lives. (This emphasizes those aspects which, as noted above, Baldwin (1993) argues should be seen as 'neighbourhood'.)

It is in this sense that community may be unreal for the person who has left a long-stay hospital; having a home of one's own may actually be isolating, and even living as part of a group may emphasize the extent to which residential provision is separated socially from the surrounding local society (Hugman, 1989). Community can be rejecting as well as accepting. Indeed, it is partly through this exclusion that the institution may be recreated in a dispersed form. Community as a description of life within group-care settings (such as a residential home or nursing home) is equally problematic, for similar reasons. There may be movement of people in and out of the building(s) identified as 'the home' but the nature of the social relations involved may be constructed around the separation of residents, their 'otherness', their needs, and not as ordinary members of the local society. Moreover, residents may be in 'a home' but not 'at home' insofar as the group context places limitations on the degree of choice and control they have over their own lives.

Community as place is distinct from home. It is the surrounding, tangible aspects of local society within which home is located. Community as shared interest is more pervasive, reflecting the sets of social relations within which each of us is a part. In this way home and community can be seen as interlocking rather than as exclusively bounded. There is a permeability, the control of which in relation to the use of care services constitutes choice, that is, when service users are able to exercise sufficient influence over decisions about people, timing, process and procedures to make use of assistance, formal and informal, so that they can live their lives within the local society on a comparable basis to others around them. It is under these circumstances that the links between home and community are likely to be seen as positive.

What, then, is care in the community?

In this discussion the meaning of care has been held to embrace a number of factors. Chiefly it has been seen as commitment to people, the ideas that are important to them and to their needs. Tied to this has been the notion that the expression of commitment to people's needs is through the provision of appropriate forms of assistance which recognize both the location (social spaces, structures) and social relations within which people live. Care is both the accomplishment of the practical tasks which enable this to occur (caring for, labour) and the expression of intent to promote the good of the person who requires assistance (caring about, love). At a neighbourhood level, as opposed to in the home, these factors are not always clear. The debates which have been considered, around gender and the family in particular, arise from the way in which some communities of interest dominate others. For community care to be more of a reality there would need to be a greater sense that the members of society, locally and nationally, can express commitment to all fellow citizens beyond sectional interests. In other words, it would require there to be a bridge between the coincidence of residence and the difference of interests through which each person might feel 'in community' only with some others.

This understanding draws on a Rawlsian approach to questions of social justice (for example, see Barry, 1990). That is, it is based on a framework by which the appropriateness of social arrangements to promote welfare would be determined by bracketing out sectional interests. In this formulation inequalities are acceptable only insofar as they promote the interests of those who are most disadvantaged. Community care on such a basis would be the formulation of practices and policies which promote choice and control for people who require assistance and support in daily life, without oppressing other groups. (There are parallels here with the idea of a welfare society discussed by Robson (1976), although I am stressing the local level at which it is directly experienced. The links are in the idea that civil society as distinct from the state may care through policies and structures.)

In a divided and oppressive society, therefore, the possibility of community care may seem to be remote. Unless the interests of women, black and ethnic minority people, disabled people and other oppressed groups are recognized and responded to positively then community care will continue to mean the fragmented provision of assistance and support to people in settings which only approximate to a home environment. This would necessitate an acceptance of diversity that would not be easy. The securing of equality within diversity is possibly the greatest challenge that faces any attempt to promote social justice in welfare.

The promotion of care which relates to local communities and which succeeds in overcoming the dichotomy of caring for and caring about would also necessitate a recognition of the reality of current social patterns and continuing change. Allan (1983) summarizes the evidence that although families continue to undertake the vast bulk of caring work, the networks of informal relations that may be said to constitute local 'communities' frequently do not contribute to this work. Indeed, as noted above, the act of caring may cause them to fracture or wither. Also, it is important that the changes continuing to take place in families and communities be acknowledged (Edgar, 1992). Already there is an increased number of families that have been reconstituted during the lifecourse of their members, and the easy assumptions in contemporary community care policies about connections between family, care and community simply will not be sustainable. Most importantly, the lives of women simply cannot be assumed to be the pliable material of social policy, as has so often been the case. There is no further 'reserve army of caring labour' waiting to be drafted (Davis and Ellis, 1995; Finch, 1989). Policies which are designed on this assumption can serve only to perpetuate gender oppression in this regard.

As an alternative, professionals and policy-makers might be well advised to be engaged in the task of helping to develop services which are grounded in the reality of daily life for people who require care support. Baldwin (1993), in arguing for the 'neighbourhood' approach, stresses not only the local nature of the model but also that it would require a shift in the thinking and practice of the professionals. It may well be that these sectional interests, along with policy imperatives to control social welfare expenditure, are major barriers to more responsive services or practices in which service users can engage in open dialogue with professionals (Hugman, 1991). There is little evidence in any of the advanced industrial countries that community care is moving in that direction, although there are many small independent projects which have greater success (Warner, 1991). Were that to be achieved on a larger scale then it might be possible to speak of care in community. At present, however, this continues to be more of a hope than a reality.

Acknowledgements

I would like to acknowledge the critical support of Steve Baldwin and Moira Peelo in their comments on an earlier version of this chapter.

References

Allan, G. 1983: 'Informal networks of care: issues raised by Barclay' in *British Journal of Social Work* **13**(4), 417–34.

Arber, S. and Gilbert, N. 1989: Men: the forgotten carers. *Sociology* **23**(1), 111–18.

Baldwin, S. 1993: *The myth of community care: an alternative neighbourhood model of care.* London: Chapman & Hall.

Barry, N. 1990: *Welfare.* Buckingham: Open University Press.

Brandon, D. 1991: The implications of normalisation work. In Ramon, S. (ed.), *Beyond community care.* Basingstoke/London: Macmillan Education/MIND, 35–55.

Bryan, D., Dadzie, S. and Scafe, S. 1985: *The heart of the race.* London: Virago.

Bryson, L. 1992: *Welfare and the state.* Basingstoke: Macmillan Education.

Bulmer, M. 1987: *The social basis of community care.* Hemel Hempstead: Allen and Unwin.

Dalley, G. 1988: *Ideologies of caring.* London: Macmillan.

Davis, A. and Ellis, K. 1995: Enforced altruism in community care. In Hugman, R. and Smith, D. (eds), *Ethical issues in social work.* London: Routledge, 136–54.

DHSS 1982: *Growing older,* Cmnd 8173, Department of Health and Social Security. London: HMSO.

Edgar, D. 1992: Constructing social care: the Australian dilemma. In Close, P. (ed.), *The state and caring.* Basingstoke: Macmillan Education.

Finch, J. 1989: *Family obligations and social change.* Cambridge: Polity Press.

Finch, J. and Groves, D. 1980: Community care and the family: a case for equal opportunities? *Journal of Social Policy* **9**(4), 487–514.

Fisher, M. 1994: Man-made care: community care and older male carers. *British Journal of Social Work* **24**(6), 659–80.

Goffman, E. 1968: *Asylums.* Harmondsworth: Penguin Books.

Graham, H. 1983: Caring: a labour of love. In Finch, J. and Groves, D. (eds), *A labour of love.* London: Routledge and Kegan Paul, 13–30.

Gunaratnam, Y. 1993: Asian carers in Britain. In Bornat, J. Pereira, C. Pilgrim, D. and Williams, F. (eds), *Community care: a reader.* Basingstoke: Macmillan Education, 114–23.

Henrard, J.-C. 1991: Care for elderly people in the European Community. *Social Policy and Administration* **25**(3), 184–92.

Home and Community Care Act 1985: Canberra: Australian Government Publishing Service.

Hugman, R. 1989: Rehabilitation and community care in mental health 2: aspects of care in the community. *Practice* **3**(3), 199–214.

Hugman, R. 1991: *Power in caring professions.* Basingstoke: Macmillan Education.

Hugman, R. 1994: *Ageing and the care of older people in Europe.* Basingstoke: Macmillan Education.

Jani-le Bris, H. 1992: *Pris en charge familiale des dependents ages.* Paris/Dublin:

CLEIRPPA/European Foundation for the Improvement of Living and Working Conditions.

McDowell, D., Barniskis, L. and Wright, S. 1990: The Wisconsin community options program: planning and packaging long term support for individuals. In Howe, A. Ozanne, E. and Selby Smith, C. (eds), *Community care policy and practice*. Clayton, Vic.: Monash University Press.

Macfarlane, A. 1993: The right to make choices. In Bornat, J. Pereira, C. Pilgrim, D. and Williams, F. (eds), *Community care: a reader*. Basingstoke: Macmillan Education, 335–37.

McLeay, L.J. 1982: *In a home or at home: accommodation and home care for the aged*. Canberra: Australian Government Publishing Service.

Mayeroff, M. 1972: *On caring*. New York: Harper and Row.

Means, R. and Smith, R. 1994: *Community care: policy and practice*. Basingstoke: Macmillan Education.

Morris, J. 1991: *Pride against prejudice: transforming attitudes to disability*. London: The Women's Press.

Murphy, E. 1991: *After the asylums: community care for people with mental illness*. London: Faber & Faber.

National Health Service and Community Care Act 1990: *Public general acts – Elizabeth II* chapter 19. London: HMSO.

NISW 1982: *Social workers, their role and tasks*. The Barclay Report, National Institute for Social Work. London: Bedford Square Press.

Nisbet, R.A. 1966: *The sociological tradition*. New York: Basic Books.

Ozanne, E. 1990: Development of Australian health and social policy in relation to the aged and the emergence of home care services. In Howe, A. Ozanne, E. and Selby Smith, C. (eds), *Community care policy and practice*. Clayton, Vic.: Monash University Press, 8–24.

Pereira, C. 1993: Anthology: the breadth of community. In Bornat, J. Pereira, C. Pilgrim, D. and Williams, F. (eds), *Community care: a reader*. Basingstoke: Macmillan Education, 5–21.

Perrin, B. and Nirje, B. 1989: Setting the record straight: a critique of some frequent misconceptions of the normalisation principle. In Brechin, A. and Walmsley, J. (eds), *Making connections*. London: Hodder & Stoughton, 220–28.

Rapley, M. and Baldwin, S. 1995: Normalisation – metatheory or metaphysics? A conceptual critique. *Australia and New Zealand Journal of Developmental Disabilities* **20**(2), 141–57.

Redfield, R. 1960: *The little community/peasant society and culture*. Chicago, IL: Phœnix Books.

Robson, W.A. 1976: *Welfare state and welfare society: illusion and reality*. London: Allen and Unwin.

Roche, M. 1992: Rethinking citizenship: welfare, ideology and change in modern society. Cambridge: Polity Press.

Scull, A. 1979: *Museums of madness*. London: Allen Lane.

Scull, A. 1984: *Decarceration*, 2nd edition. Cambridge: Polity Press.

Ungerson, C. 1983: Why do women care? In Finch, J. and Groves, D. (eds), *A labour of love*. London: Routledge and Kegan Paul.

Ungerson, C. 1990: The language of care. In Ungerson, C. (ed.), *Gender and caring: work and welfare in Britain and Scandinavia*. Hemel Hempstead: Harvester Wheatsheaf, 31–49.

Warner, R. 1991: Creative programming. In Ramon, S. (ed.), *Beyond community care.* Basingstoke/London: Macmillan Education/MIND, 114–35.

Wolfensberger, W. and Tullman, S. 1989: A brief outline of the principle of normalisation. In Brechin, A. and Walmsley, J. (eds), *Making connections.* London: Hodder and Stoughton, 211–19.

Index